"Life will never be perfect, but *Help in a Hurry* gives you the tools to navigate the messy moments with grace and resilience. Dr. Leaf's wisdom and compassionate guidance are immensely valuable for anyone seeking practical, research-backed advice on how to transform overwhelming thoughts into purposeful growth."

Demi-Leigh Tebow, former Miss Universe, bestselling author, entrepreneur, and speaker

"Life can be overwhelming, and at times it feels like the weight of the world is too much to bear. But what if we could learn to carry that weight with more grace? This book is a powerful guide for anyone looking to better understand themselves, manage the chaos of life, and cultivate a healthier mindset. It's not just about surviving—it's about thriving. With raw honesty and practical wisdom, this book reminds us that healing is a process, and each step forward counts. If you're seeking peace, clarity, and the strength to keep going, I can't recommend this enough."

Michelle Williams, actress, author, and mental health advocate

"Everyone has intrusive thoughts, overthinking, and stress from being around difficult people. It's harder now than it's ever been. Dr. Leaf's book masterfully shows you what's really going on with your stress and what to do about it, based on real science and her decades of clinical experience. It's a must-read if you want to thrive instead of just getting by every single day!"

Dave Asprey, father of biohacking and four-time *New York Times* bestselling author

"Dr. Leaf's latest book not only provides deep understanding but also offers practical strategies for overcoming everyday challenges and building mental resilience. An essential read for anyone looking to foster inner strength and navigate the journey toward emotional well-being as they face the ups and downs of life."

Dr. Josh Axe, DC, DNM, CNS

"Dr. Leaf gets it. Life is messy, but *Help in a Hurry* reminds us that we don't have to figure it out alone. This book is a timely and practical gift for navigating tough moments."

Judah Smith, pastor of Churchome and author of *Jesus Is*

"Dr. Caroline Leaf's *Help in a Hurry* is the perfect toolkit for navigating life's messiest moments. Packed with quick, science-backed strategies, it's an empowering reminder that healing and growth are always within reach—even in the stormiest seasons."

Dr. Will Cole, leading functional medicine expert, *New York Times* bestselling author, and host of *The Art of Being Well* podcast

"What if you had tools to help you get through life's most difficult moments right at your fingertips? I'm beyond grateful that Dr. Leaf created *Help in a Hurry*. These tools are simple, practical, backed by science, and just flat-out work!"

Shawn Stevenson, bestselling author of *Eat Smarter* and *Eat Smarter Family Cookbook*

"In Dr. Caroline Leaf's *Help in a Hurry*, she combines her brilliant scientific mind with her big heart, brimming with compassionate care and wisdom, to create a uniquely practical and effective guide that is very much needed in today's hurried world."

Kimberly Snyder, three-time *New York Times* bestselling author of *The Hidden Power of the Five Hearts*

"Life is messy—there's no sugarcoating it. This book is an incredible roadmap for anyone who wants to take control of their mental well-being, find balance, and feel more at peace. It's filled with practical advice, real-life wisdom, and the kind of uplifting inspiration we all need when life feels like it's getting the best of us. We can't pour from an empty cup, and this book is the perfect reminder that prioritizing mental well-being isn't a luxury; it's essential. I can't recommend it enough."

Alli Webb, founder of Drybar and Messy and *New York Times* and *USA Today* bestselling author

"A masterpiece in finding calm amid life's chaos, scheduling specific times to worry, and reminding ourselves that sometimes it's okay to not be okay. Dr. Leaf articulates beautifully the difference between peace and happiness, and she leaves the reader with tangible nuggets to digest and put into practice while teaching us how to reduce anxiety. A must-read."

Craig Siegel, *Wall Street Journal* bestselling author, coach, teacher, TEDx speaker, eight-time marathoner, and investor

"Dr. Caroline Leaf is one of the most prolific clinical and research neuroscientists in the world; she is also a phenomenal human who genuinely cares about people. This book presents the best of what she has to offer, with practical instruction to help anyone and everyone better manage anxiety and stress. Read it and experience more peace in a hurry!"

Rory Vaden, *New York Times* bestselling author of *Take the Stairs*

"In these turbulent and stressful times, *Help in a Hurry* lets us know that true, simple, and effective tools are available. Many in today's world are struggling daily to navigate life's messiness and chaos, too often experiencing anxiousness, overwhelm, energy drain, and stress-related physiological symptoms. This book is filled with practical tips and tools, which when applied simply and briefly—yet consistently—will result in gradual change into a life of increasing inner calm. Small, steady steps according to these practical strategies offer a way through and a way out of inner turmoil, self-hatred, and living focused on the past or future. We can learn not to regret the past nor wish to shut the door on it; we can also gradually learn to not get stuck in 'future tripping' that sabotages our living in the today we each have been given. Progress, not perfection, is the goal. Thank you, Dr. Leaf, for bringing us yet another actionable, evidence-based, and timely book!"

Robert P. Turner, MD, MSCR, QEEGD, BCN

HELP IN A HURRY

HELP IN A HURRY

SIMPLE TIPS FOR FINDING PEACE WHEN YOU'RE OVERWHELMED, ANXIOUS, OR STRESSED

DR. CAROLINE LEAF

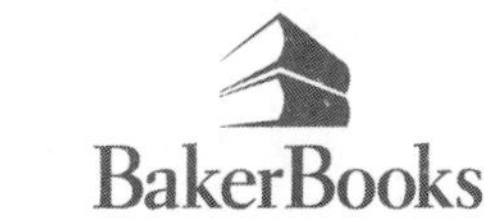

a division of Baker Publishing Group
Grand Rapids, Michigan

Published by Baker Books
a division of Baker Publishing Group
Grand Rapids, Michigan
www.bakerbooks.com

Printed in the United States of America

Library of Congress Cataloging-in-Publication Data
Names: Leaf, Caroline, 1963– author
Title: Help in a hurry : simple tips for finding peace when you're overwhelmed, anxious, or stressed / Dr. Caroline Leaf.
Description: Grand Rapids, Michigan : Baker Books, a division of Baker Publishing Group, [2025] | Includes bibliographical references.
Identifiers: LCCN 2025000073 | ISBN 9780801093265 (cloth) | ISBN 9781540905307 (paperback) | ISBN 9781493407828 (ebook)
Subjects: LCSH: Stress management—Popular works | Self-care, Health—Popular works.
Classification: LCC RA785 .L433 2025 | DDC 155.9/042—dc23/eng/20250312
LC record available at https://lccn.loc.gov/2025000073

This publication is intended to provide helpful and informative material on the subjects addressed. Readers should consult their personal health professionals before adopting any of the suggestions in this book or drawing inferences from it. The author and publisher expressly disclaim responsibility for any adverse effects arising from the use or application of the information contained in this book.

Cover design by Emily Weigel

Baker Publishing Group publications use paper produced from sustainable forestry practices and postconsumer waste whenever possible.

25 26 27 28 29 30 31 7 6 5 4 3 2 1

My sweet Alexy,
your candle burned out way too soon,
but the people you touched still feel its warmth
because your candle was bright
and burned hard and fast for those you loved.

Contents

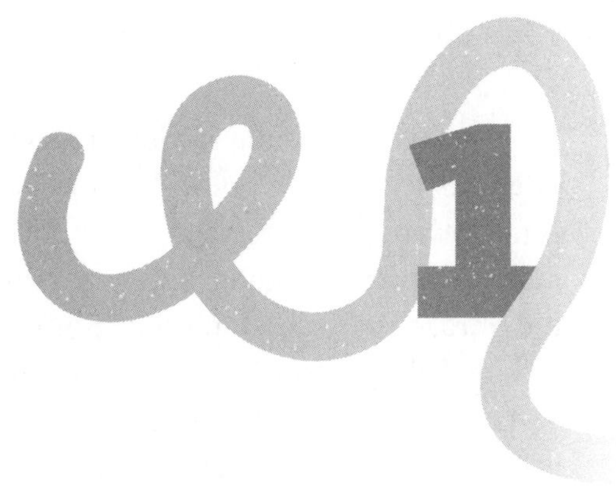

Help in a Hurry, What's That?

Are any of these phrases a part of your daily routine?

> "I've had it up to here!"
> "I can't take it anymore."
> "My head's about to explode."
> "Give me strength!"
> "I give up!"
> "Why me?"
> "I am at the end of my rope."
> "I am going to tear my hair out!"
> "I am at a breaking point."
> "I am sick with worry."
> "I am an anxious wreck."
> "This was the straw that broke the camel's back."
> "I am climbing the walls!"
> "It's all downhill from here."

We all have "off" days, where everything that can go wrong does. As the saying goes, "When it rains, it pours." If you think about it, we have a lot of these kinds of sayings, in many different languages. My personal favorite is the Arabic phrase that translates as, "Some days honey, some days onions." The idea of a bad day is pretty universal!

This doesn't mean, however, that we have to stand in the rain without an umbrella or raincoat. This is why I wrote this book: While "bad days" are universal, knowing what to do when we are faced with the ups and downs of life is *not*. So many of us find ourselves at a loss when [insert your favorite bad word here] hits the fan. We know that bad things happen but not *what to do* when they happen.

This book is filled with simple, quick strategies to assist you when things are going badly and you are at a loss for what to do. It's basically a guide to dealing with those "stormy," "oniony" days, based on my own personal and professional experience, my work in the field of mental health for over three decades, and what the latest research is telling us about how to manage our mind and brain to build up our mental resilience.

Sure, we can go through life from crisis to crisis and sort of make up things as we go along. The problem with this approach to "bad days" is that the more we just let things happen, the more we are allowing these things to shape us rather than using the bad times as opportunities to learn, grow, and build up our strength so that we are not so easily swayed by the vicissitudes of life.

Just think of a recent time when you got irritated. If you remained in that irritated state of mind, there's a good chance it progressed and spread like a virus into other parts of your day, blocking access to your mental resilience and making the small things seem so much worse, while handicapping your ability to deal with major life stressors. And, if you get into a pattern of reacting this way, in 63 days it becomes a habit that can severely impact your well-being and make you feel so much worse in the short- and long-term.

Note I said **63 days**, which is roughly the time it takes to form a habit.[1] This means that we *do* have some wiggle room to prevent something we are doing from becoming a habit that drives us and influences our mental and physical health. We have time to choose how to react rather than letting what happens to us determine our resilience to life. This is what this book is all about: how to get help in a hurry, develop good habits that build up your resilience, and figure out a game plan for life, which is, inevitably, a very messy affair.

So, in this book we have rainstorms, onions, and viruses—and what to do about them. What you will not find is the promise that things will always be okay or *x* number of steps guaranteed to take away your pain, stress, and irritation and make you happy all the time. It is not a book about optimizing your life to make all your dreams come true or to help you live till you are 120.

There are a lot of books out there on these topics, and you may or may not find them helpful. I, personally, find many of them a little overwhelming, and I know I am not alone. There have been many times in life when I needed a helping hand that told me it's okay not to be okay and it's okay to take life one step at a time and just figure out how to make it through the next hour, day, or week—and this is what you will find here: a helping hand, free of judgment, because who even has time for that? In these pages, it is all about figuring out how to manage the mind and emotions amid the day-to-day chaos of life. It is simply about being *okay*, because so many of us are struggling with just that.

Of course, many of these struggles are deeply rooted in trauma and past experiences that take time and a lot of work to learn how to manage, which I discuss in detail in my previous books, my Neurocycle app, and my research.[2] This book, on the other hand, focuses on strategies to help you survive those storms that just rush in—those unexpected, and sometimes expected, struggles that cut your legs out from under you and leave you dazed and not sure how to get up.

In fact, this is an important part of any healing journey: We need to learn how to *get through the next moment* before we can dive in and do all the necessary healing journey work. So, see this book as a resource, something on tap to help you when you are in a hurry and have a lot going on. It is filled with strategies to teach you how to steady your mind and focus in the midst of chaos so that you can get from A to B. It is not a comprehensive guide to the healing journey but rather will help you stay on the path so you can do the rest of the work and live your best, most fulfilled life.

It is important to note that the tips and strategies in this book are not quick fixes or final solutions. They are designed to help you get through the day without falling apart because you are stressed out or overwhelmed and to get you to the point where you are able to work on your issues and trauma in order to rewrite your story. So, if you notice that some of these scenarios *are* pretty strong patterns in your life and you are taking a little longer than anticipated to really make the changes you want, don't be disheartened. As mentioned, it does take at least 63 days to change a habit, and this is something you are more than capable of over time and with help.

And this starts with accepting that it's okay not to be okay, as mentioned above, and that it's okay for life to be chaotic and messy from time to time, as long as we don't stay stuck in the "bad day" zone.

It is about taking those onions and making something of them rather than letting them bring us to tears; it is about putting on our coat and rain boots and grabbing our umbrella so that the storm doesn't wash us away; it is about building up our immunity to that virus so that it doesn't set us down for days, weeks, or months.

The guides in this book are ways to exit that reactive mode where we make choices we end up regretting or build habits in the moment that end up hurting us. It's about preparing properly today so we don't have to do as much *repairing* tomorrow!

In the next chapter, I will start by giving you a little bit of the science behind how the mind-brain-body connection works, what happens when we struggle with the ups and downs of life, and why it's okay not to be okay and what we can do about this. Then I will go through some of the major issues many of us face as we go through life, giving you practical tips, examples, and strategies to teach you how to cope in the moment, get through the day, and move on to bigger and brighter things!

To download the Neurocycle app, visit www.neurocycle.app

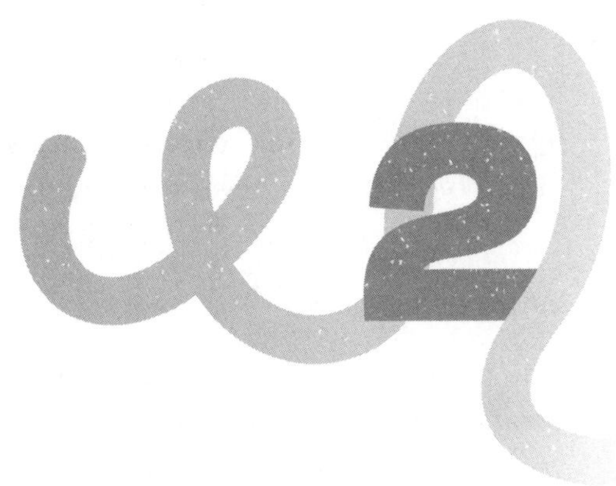

Help, What's Going On in My Head?

When everything around us feels like it is a mess, it is easy to imagine that our mind and brain are too. Think of words and phrases like "scatterbrained," "brain fog," "mind-boggling," "drive you out of your mind," "go mental," and "brain fried." Everything feels out of control outside of our head, so it must be the same inside it, right?

Here, it helps to understand what exactly goes on in the mind, brain, and body when we experience life and why things feel so messy inside our head when we are stressed, overwhelmed, and need "help in a hurry."

We don't have to remember all these facts when we are struggling, but knowing what is going on and how we can change how we respond to life can be incredibly helpful. The big picture helps us step outside of ourselves so we don't get so lost in all the craziness of life that we forget there is always hope. It is never too late to change our mind and positively impact how we think, feel, and choose—and how this plays out in our life. It is never too late to get help in a hurry!

What Is the Mind?

The mind can be a tricky concept, so it's best to start with what the mind is *not*. Your mind is not your brain, just as you are not your brain. The mind is separate, yet inseparable from, the brain. The mind uses the brain, and the brain responds to the mind. The brain doesn't produce the mind. Yes, there would be no conscious experience without the brain, but experience cannot be reduced to the brain's actions.

The mind is energy, and it generates energy through thinking, feeling, and choosing. That means we generate energy through our mind-in-action 24/7, which is part of the activity we pick up with brain technology. When we generate this mind energy through thinking, feeling, and choosing, we build *thoughts*, which are physical structures in our brain. This building of thoughts is called *neuroplasticity*, or the ability of the brain to change.

The mind is a stream of nonconscious and conscious activity when we're awake and a stream of nonconscious activity when we're asleep. It's characterized by a triad of thinking, feeling, and choosing. When we think, we will feel, and when we think and feel, we will choose. These three aspects work together.

You have a unique way you think, feel, and choose, which is your *identity*. When your thinking, feeling, and choosing are off for some reason, this will affect your identity. When you think, feel, and choose, you create, and this creation is a *thought*.

And you're always thinking, feeling, and choosing! When you're awake, you think and feel and choose to build thoughts. When you're asleep, you sort out the thoughts you've built during the day.

What Is the Brain?

The brain is an extremely complex *neuroplastic responder*. This essentially means that each time it's stimulated by the mind, it responds in many different ways, including making neurochemical, genetic, and electromagnetic changes. These, in turn, grow and change structures in the brain, building or wiring in new physical thoughts.

So, the brain is not the producer of the mind but rather the filter of the mind.

The brain is never the same because it changes with every experience we have, every moment of every day. And we can learn how to control this with our unique thinking, feeling, and choosing. We can use our mind to change our brain, which is what you will be learning how to do using the "help in a hurry" tips in this book.

The Three Parts of the Mind

The mind is divided into the conscious mind, the nonconscious mind, and the subconscious mind. To understand these three parts, think of a tree. The top of the tree is the *conscious* mind, which is our communication and behavior, or what we say and do.

The tree trunk area and the grass around it are the *subconscious* mind, or the prompts from the nonconscious mind that are just on the edge of our conscious awareness. These are those tip-of-the-tongue, can't-quite-put-your-finger-on-it cues that evoke and trigger that feeling that something needs to be addressed—something is trying to get our attention.

The roots are the *nonconscious* mind, which is the deep, spiritual, and phenomenally fast quantum world where our truth value, intelligence, wisdom, meaning, and thoughts with their embedded memories are stored in a swirling mass of energy.

Understanding these divisions of the mind will help us better understand our mind and ourselves, which will equip us to manage what happens to us in the best way possible. When we understand the why, the how becomes so much easier!

What's in a Thought?

Thoughts are the active ingredients as well as the products of the mind. The mind converts all our experiences all day long into thoughts and builds these thoughts into the brain and body as protein tree-like structures in the brain and hedge-like structures in the body cells. Thoughts are the accumulation of all our experiences, how we view and process each moment, and are pretty much what drives us. They also become part of our entire physical being as these protein structures, which hold our memory.

Each thought also has corresponding electrochemical reactions in our brain and body. When we think, energy and chemicals course through our brain and body in magnificently complex electromagnetic waves and electrochemical feedback loops, which, if we could hear them, would sound like the most exquisite orchestral symphony if they are healthy thoughts or earsplitting cacophony if they are toxic.

What Is a Memory?

Thoughts are made of memories. In the brain, these physical thought structures grow from the tops of neurons as clusters of branches called *dendrites*, which look like trees. A thought can have from a few hundred memories to thousands of memories. This is why some thoughts can be so overwhelming; as a thought comes into the conscious mind, it opens like a flower blooming, the memories pouring out like pollen in springtime. If this is a good memory, you may find yourself flooded with happy feelings. If this is a toxic memory or trauma, well, it is kind of like having really bad allergies from all that pollen flying about that you just can't get rid of. You can find yourself replaying past scenarios, creating endless "if only, would have, should have, could have" scenarios and getting stuck in the pain and discomfort of what happened to you—hence you may need help in a hurry!

Thoughts Grow from "Seeds" Like Trees and Hedges

Just like trees and hedges start growing from seeds and then develop roots, trunks, branches, and leaves, so our thoughts originate from "seeds of experiences"—our stories—and expand into numerous roots, trunks, branches, and leaves in the mind, brain, and body.

The roots are the various memories or the details of the experience. For example, the thought may be of a traumatic relationship with a family member, and all the details of the experience are the memories of the thought. Or the thought could be a really happy one of a family member, and the details of this happy thought are the memories.

The trunk symbolizes the unique way you think about and process the "root" memories of the experience. You also process each new experience through the eyes of existing thoughts with their embedded memories, which are your past experiences, to understand it better. This is your past influencing your present.

The branches reflect how this is playing out and showing up within the current context of your life and how it affects how you feel and see life, what you say and do, and how this all feels in your body. For example, as you recall the toxic thought about a problematic family member, you may feel anxious, get a stomachache, withdraw a little, and see the relationship as hopeless.

Thoughts Are Stored in Three Places

Thoughts are stored in three places: the mind, the brain, and every cell of the body. They form a connected network across your mind, brain, and body. A useful analogy to try to understand this network is to visualize your mind as the sky and thoughts as clouds in the sky, kind of like your own personal "iCloud" hovering over the thought trees in your brain and body. The mind "sky" essentially builds your experience into your personalized iCloud and then plants this experience into the brain as "thought trees" and in the body as "hedges."

The sky is all your energy combined into a single, unified living "thing" that never dies. And, just like the sky is all around you, your mind is all around you. The clouds, as your thoughts, are specific patterns made from memory particles that come from all the experiences you have had, are having, or will have. Just as you have different thoughts, so you have different cloud types and formations, and they keep changing as the weather of the mind shifts based on your experiences of life. You are constantly updating and backing up your personal iCloud sky with each new experience you have every moment of every day, just like the sky and weather always change, affecting the plants below them.

The Mind-Brain-Body Connection

Thoughts with their complex root and branch memories are not just stored in the brain; they are stored throughout the 50–100 trillion cells in the brain and body *and* in the clouds of your mind, which is why, when you are under toxic stress, for example, your heart gets "sore" or your gut gurgles and swells up—or why, when someone says something to you that triggers you, you get overwhelmed with nausea or feelings of being "sick to your stomach."

As mentioned above, the mind is how we uniquely think, feel, and choose as we go through life. The brain and body are the filter through which the mind works and, while it works, it changes our brain and body structurally as well as how they function. This mind-brain-body relationship is called *psychoneurobiology*.

One of the ways we can "see" mind energy showing up in the brain is as brain waves. Our brain waves are active all the time because the mind is always active and pushing life through our brain and body. Our brain waves change in terms of how they move through the brain, which is based on what we are thinking, doing, and feeling. When we feel tired, slow, sluggish, or dreamy and are not able to process information or emotions very well, slower brain waves are dominant. When we feel wired or hyperalert, like there is just too much going on in our brain, the higher brain wave frequencies are dominant. When we manage our mind, we are balancing these extremes, and this is different for each of us.

How our brain waves function and our daily experience of the world are inseparable because the mind *moves through the brain*, and the brain *responds to the mind*. When our emotions are out of balance or very negative (like when we aren't rising to the challenge and building new knowledge into our brain daily, or when we are responding in chaotic and reactive ways to the chronic and acute stressors of life), this will be reflected in our physiology (blood, hormones, and so on) and in our brain waves, which will be out of balance. There is a corresponding relationship between the mind and brain that plays out in our mental, emotional, neurological, and physical health.

Managing Our Mind

The connectivity and balance that the mind, brain, and body crave can be disrupted when we don't manage our mind properly. Because of the neuroplasticity of the brain, if we aren't changing our reactions to the stress, then we are reinforcing them—they don't just go away. Whatever we think about the most will grow.

If we choose to stay in a negative state of mind, this can create a toxic response in the brain that can impact every system in the brain and body. The converse also applies; if we choose to start seeing every opportunity as a chance to learn, grow, and overcome, and we find the positive in the negative, our hope starts coming back and we can positively affect our brain waves and body—down to the cellular level![1]

Why Do We Need Help in a Hurry?

This is why learning to manage our mind in the moment is so important. It teaches us how *not* to reinforce negative patterns that can hurt our mental well-being, health, and longevity.

Indeed, we all have to learn how to catch and edit our thoughts and reactions before they trigger toxic chain reactions and become ingrained neural networks, a.k.a. bad habits. In essence, you are your mind, and your mind runs your brain and body, so a messy, unmanaged mind means a messy, unmanaged brain and body, and when these three are a mess, our life can feel like a mess!

This managing, however, is easier said than done, especially when it feels like your life is falling apart around you. Hence the need for a quick helping hand in the moment, which this book aims to be, to get you through those times when everything is going wrong and your brain is about to explode.

As you practice these tips, you will quite literally be building an insurance policy into your mind-brain-body network that will open the door to your unlimited resilience, changing your mind, brain, and body for the better!

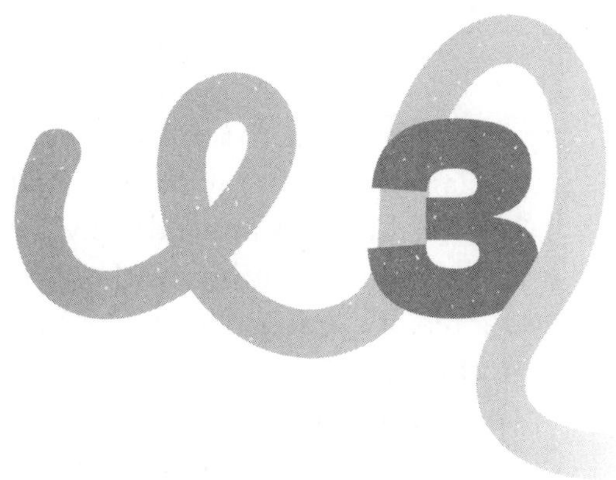

Help, I'm Under Pressure!

Pressure cookers are great. They are a one-pot wonder; you just put everything in, leave it for a bit, and voila! A delicious and nutritious meal is ready with minimal preparation or mess.

People, however, are not one-pot wonders. Life is complex. Sometimes things go well under pressure, and sometimes things go badly—especially when we are putting undue amounts of pressure on ourselves to look or act in a certain way or achieve certain things.

Of course, not all pressure is bad. We actually do pretty well under what I call "positive pressure" because it keeps us in a state of good stress (yes, there is such a thing!), which enhances rather than diminishes our performance. Think of the kind of stress you feel when you need to get something done within a certain time period, like a task, exam, or project. Good stress helps us stay alert and focused in the moment. It dilates the blood vessels around our heart, pumping blood and oxygen into our brain, and releases neurotransmitters that all work together to help us think with clarity and react in the best way possible.

We wouldn't get much done without this kind of stress. It is like an invigorating workout for the mind, brain, and body. Yes, it requires some work and effort, but afterward we feel so good!

Positive pressure helps us tap into this kind of "get things done" energy. In the past, it helped our ancestors survive, learn, develop their skills, and grow. Likewise, today it helps us survive *and* thrive. Just think of a recent time where you struggled to learn something new or achieve a certain goal, and how, even though it was stressful at times, you learned so much and unlocked another life level!

Negative pressure starts building when we get into a habit of thinking in certain ways, which twists this kind of positive pressure into a force that shifts us into a state of toxic stress. For example, feeling restless, having a hovering sense of anxiety or an underlying sense that things that brought you joy don't bring joy anymore, experiencing increased irritability and angry outbursts, and feeling tired all the time—these are all potential signs of burnout and negative stress.

This creates a lot of confusion and chaotic energy on a physiological level, upsetting the balance (*homeostasis*) between the mind, brain, and body that is intrinsic to our well-being. It drains our mental and physical energy, often leaving us feeling burned out and overwhelmed, and, if left unmanaged, can leave us vulnerable to all sorts of mental and physical issues.

Prolonged periods of this kind of stress, for example, can affect our ability to digest food and sleep, while laying the foundation for mental issues such as persistent anxiety and depression. It is therefore vital that we recognize when our body is in toxic stress so we can quickly move out of the "danger zone."

Indeed, if we consistently experience high levels of stress without taking steps to manage or reduce it, exhaustion will eventually take over, leaving us emotionally and physically burned out. We will begin to feel less motivated, since it seems like nothing we do matters, while even the smallest tasks can leave us feeling overwhelmed and broken.

Here, it is helpful to remember what pressure is. If you recall from your school days, pressure is a force. When applied to certain things, it works great. Let's go back to the pressure cooker example: This kitchen appliance traps steam through boiling water, using this pressure to increase the temperature to cook the food inside it, decreasing cooking time and increasing flavor (through less evaporation).[1] If, however, you keep this appliance cooking past the recommended time, it will eventually explode, and your kitchen will not look too great. The key is managing the pressure, limiting the cooking time, and keeping an eye on the process, much like many things in life!

Another great example of this is using an inflatable pool toy or kayak. Just enough pressure allows us to enjoy the water; too much pressure makes things go pop and can ruin a good day under the sun.

Yes, life is more complicated than appliances or pool toys, and we cannot always control the amount of pressure we are exposed to. We can, however, learn how to manage this pressure when we are the ones directing the force, and we can learn to let some steam escape when things get too hot to handle.

Pressure has to go somewhere, and we can learn how to direct it in the moment, turning our biggest assets into something that energizes rather than overwhelms us. Here are seven simple ways you can do this when it feels like everything is about to explode under pressure.

1. How to Deal with "I Didn't Get *X* Done."

Often, we put a lot of pressure on ourselves to get a certain amount of things done in a day, and if we fail to tick everything off our list, we can feel pretty stressed out, overwhelmed, and anxious.

This is something I really tend to battle with. That panicky feeling that sets in when the end of the day approaches and you realize you haven't conquered your "to-do list," and all you can think about is everything you haven't accomplished and how much of a failure you are . . . I've definitely been there, done that, got the T-shirt (or a whole collection of them).

This kind of thinking is so easy to fall into because we all have so much on our plates. It often takes just one failed task or responsibility to throw the whole day off and leave us feeling like we haven't gotten anything done at all.

When you find yourself falling into this pattern, a key thing to remember is that this is just *one* perspective. Yes, you didn't get something done; there is no denying that. But you are just focusing on *what you haven't done* instead of *what you have done*. This may sound like nitpicking, but it's a small shift that makes a world of difference when it comes to how much pressure you are under and what kind of stress state you end up in.

When you catch yourself thinking this way, the best thing you can do is pause, take some time to say out loud or write down what you have achieved, and remind yourself that there will be time to get other things done tomorrow. The more you practice this, the more you will find it becomes your default perspective when you feel under pressure rather than the "I haven't done *x*" way of thinking.

The simple table below can be used to help you track yourself doing this and your progress. This is optional, but it can be really helpful if you want to practice shifting your perspective and making this new way of thinking a habit!

The first column is what I call a mindhack: something simple you can do in the moment to get your neurophysiology under control and help you calm down your mind, brain, and body so you can think more clearly. Essentially, a mindhack will help you shift into a good state of stress. This can be anything from a breathing exercise to a physical activity to a grounding exercise; do whatever works for you when you feel the pressure building.

The second column is the pressure statement you find yourself saying in the moment—the "I haven't done *x*." When you write it down, it loses a lot of its power over you. Writing also helps you become more objective and analytical, almost like a friend is telling you that this is how they react and asking you for your advice. It allows you to stand outside yourself and really think about your thinking, feeling, and reacting.

The third column is where you examine how your perception is affecting you mentally or physically. It is where you think about how the negative pressure of "I didn't get *x* done" is putting you in a state of negative stress. For example, is your perception making you feel stressed, anxious, or upset? Do you feel sick to your stomach?

The fourth column is what I call the mindshift, where you reframe your thinking. It is the "How can I see things differently and make this pressure work for me rather than against me?" section. Here, you will practice focusing on what you have accomplished rather than what you have yet to do.

You can do this quickly, in under a minute, or take as much time as you need. Below is just one example of how this can look. You can also write it down in another way that works for you or download this table with spaces to work into using the QR code at the end of the chapter.

"I Didn't Get X Done."	
Mindhack	Practice deep belly breathing for ten seconds, in and out, nice and slowly.
What am I thinking?	I haven't finished responding to all my emails! People are going to get upset!
How do I feel?	Tension in my shoulders and an upset stomach.
Mindshift	I did respond to the three really important emails in my inbox, and the other five can wait till tomorrow because they weren't actually that urgent now that I think about it. I just made them urgent because I wanted to tick them off my to-do list.

2. How to Deal with "I Have to Have It All Together."

So many of us feel like we must have it all together all the time, but the fact is that we are only human and we ALL make mistakes, mess up, and get things wrong. Feeling like we have to be perfect all the time is one of the quickest ways we can turn positive pressure into negative pressure and enter a toxic state of stress because it really is impossible! We are essentially setting ourselves up for failure every time we start thinking this way.

When you find yourself falling into this pattern of thinking, the most important thing you can do is stop and remind yourself that *no one has it all together*. Work on not comparing your life to what you feel like others are doing, because you are only seeing what they want you to see. They, too, are not perfect and are probably struggling as much as you are.

Moreover, the way you think and act, and your experiences, make you completely and utterly unique, which means you will only end up hurting yourself when you fall into the comparison trap. You will never be able to be anyone else but you, and you are amazing, even if you are not perfect all the time.

To practice this way of thinking, you can use a similar table to the one above: List out a calming exercise (the mindhack), what you are thinking when you feel like you have to have it all together, how this is affecting you mentally and physically, and how you will change the way you are thinking about this to create a good type of pressure that helps you rather than harms you (the mindshift).

As mentioned, this is optional but really helpful if you want to practice shifting your perspective and making this new way of seeing things a habit! I recommend using this table if this is an issue you have noticed in your life. Try doing it daily for about one to three weeks.

Below is just one example of how this can look. You can also write it down in another way that works for you or download this table with spaces to work into using the QR code at the end of the chapter.

"I Have to Have It All Together."	
Mindhack	Do some box breathing: Breathe in for 4 counts / hold for 4 counts / breathe out for 4 counts / breathe in for 4 counts. Repeat this as many times as necessary.
What am I thinking?	I need to have it all together because if I don't, I will fail my team/partner/children.
How do I feel?	I am worried and anxious all the time, and I am experiencing a lot of nervous heart palpitations.
Mindshift	No one has it all together! Just because that person at work or on social media seems like they get everything done and are perfect, I am only seeing part of the picture, and they are only human too!

3. How to Deal with "I Must Succeed."

It is easy to fall into the trap of thinking that we must succeed at something or achieve something to be worthy. When you feel like this, remind yourself that you define your own success! There is something you can do that no one else can do.

When you find yourself falling prey to these kinds of thoughts, practice reminding yourself of this, especially when you start falling into the comparison trap again. Once again, you can list out a calming exercise (the mindhack), what you are thinking when you feel like you have to have it all together, how this is affecting you mentally and physically, and how you will change the way you are thinking about this to create a good type of pressure that helps you rather than harms you (the mindshift).

Below is an example of how this can look. You can also write it down in another way that works for you or download this table with spaces to work into using the QR code at the end of the chapter.

"I Must Succeed."	
Mindhack	Acknowledge: 5 things you can see around you. 4 things you can touch around you. 3 things you can hear around you. 2 things you can smell around you. 1 thing you can taste near you. Now, as you breathe deeply, close your eyes and fully immerse yourself in the present moment, feeling grounded and centered in your surroundings.
What am I thinking?	I must succeed at this task. If I fail, everything will go wrong!
How do I feel?	Anxious and upset. I am snapping at everyone because I feel under pressure and am worried about what I need to do.
Mindshift	If I don't succeed at this task, this doesn't mean I am not worthy or am not a success. I can do x, and I have succeeded at *y* in the past. I define my own success, and this looks like . . .

4. How to Deal with "I Cannot Make a Mistake."

Even though we all make mistakes, it is easy to think we shouldn't mess up and we need to get things right all the time. But it is important to recognize that our failures are often as important as our successes, and they teach us important life lessons that help us grow as a person.

If you find yourself emotionally holding on to the mistakes you've made, noticing more of what you've done wrong than what you've gotten right, and getting anxious when you do a good but not perfect job, you may have fallen into the perfectionism trap, where you can't accept your own or anyone else's weaknesses.

If this sounds like you, take the time to notice when you do this and remind yourself that there is a difference between wanting to achieve certain things and thinking you need to do everything perfectly all the time. Remind yourself that mistakes and learning are part of life, and you can work hard even if you take breaks and set up self-boundaries. And, when you find yourself thinking about what you got wrong, remind yourself of what you have gotten right too!

The most important part of this process is asking yourself what this experience has taught you and focusing on how you have grown and what you have learned. In many cases, we tend to see just two options: the winner or the loser. We often do not see the third option: the learner! A great quote that helps me when I feel this way is a common adaptation of words by Thomas A. Edison, who contributed to the invention of the lightbulb and many other major technological advances in the late nineteenth and early twentieth centuries: "I have not failed. I've just found 10,000 ways that won't work."[2]

You can use the same table to help you practice this, if you want. You can also write it down in another way that works for you or download this table with spaces to work into using the QR code at the end of the chapter.

How to Deal with "I Cannot Make a Mistake."	
Mindhack	Visualize people congratulating you for what you did and what you have learned, even if you made a mistake.
What am I thinking?	I cannot mess this up; I have to do it perfectly!
How do I feel?	I feel panicky and can't concentrate. My heart rate feels fast and my palms are sweaty.
Mindshift	I now know what doesn't work; this is so great! I have learned something important that will help me in the future.

5. How to Deal with "I Will Let Everyone Down."

Sometimes, it is easy to feel like we always let people down and are just failures. Here, it is important to remind yourself that we all fail at times, as mentioned above, and that your failures help you grow as a person. Trying your best is the only way forward, even when it doesn't work out like you planned, because you will learn so much.

At the end of the day, life is pretty unpredictable. We can't always control everything to make sure things turn out well, because so much is out of our control. It is important to remember this when it feels like everything is falling apart. It is also helpful to look back at your past experiences and think about a time in your life when things didn't work out but you got through it in the end.

But it is one thing to say this and know it is true and another thing to practice it! Again, using our table is a really helpful way to do this. You can also write it down in another way that works for you or download this table with spaces to work into using the QR code at the end of the chapter.

"I Will Let Everyone Down."	
Mindhack	Stretch your arms and legs as you breathe in deeply. Do this for several minutes. Feel the tension leave your mind and body!
What am I thinking?	I am the only one who can do this task, and if I don't, I will let everyone down.
How do I feel?	I am worried and feel stressed out. My stomach is in knots, and I have a terrible headache!
Mindshift	Nothing is certain; life is unpredictable. Remember when I planned x, but things turned out very differently? It wasn't the end of the world—people didn't look at me differently or judge me harshly.

6. How to Deal with "I Feel Exhausted All the Time."

We often take on so much and expect ourselves to do so much that we quickly find ourselves stressed out, overwhelmed, and exhausted. Yes, many of us love the idea of a vacation or break, but we often feel guilty about taking even one day off. In many cases, we find ourselves in a catch-22: We have so much to do, but we can barely get through it all because we are exhausted and at our wit's end. This is one of the fastest ways to turn positive pressure into negative pressure and enter a toxic state of stress.

Giving our brain a break is essential to our productivity, efficiency, and ability to think creatively. It helps us function well under pressure and is intrinsic to that "get things done" energy we all need to harness at certain times in our life. This is why it is so important we learn when to say no and when to pause, otherwise we increase our risk for burnout and chronic health issues.

Remember, our nonconscious mind never stops. However, the conscious mind and brain *do* get tired because they work on energy. This is kind of like when we have a whole lot of apps open on our phone, the brightness is on full, and we are constantly using it—very soon the battery will die. And, like you need to recharge your phone, you also need to recharge your brain and conscious mind.

It's best we do this in a regular way, by incorporating periods of rest into our daily schedule to keep the brain charged all day long. This will also help us better know when to switch off at the end of the day. If we go for too long without rest, we may think we are okay, but the next day we won't feel as rested as we should, and we may notice our creativity or ability to think clearly is off because we didn't recharge regularly the day before and pushed the conscious mind and brain to the limit. We can quickly get into a pattern of living where we are so focused on what needs to get done that we forget how to enjoy life, which can have a serious impact on our well-being.

Indeed, when we put a lot of negative pressure on ourselves to perform a certain way or meet certain standards, it is easy to feel on edge all the time, like we are just waiting for the other shoe to drop and to make a mistake, repeating the vicious circle of negative pressure and toxic stress.

If this sounds familiar, do a lifestyle check and ask yourself:

- Do I take enough breaks to recharge?
- Do I give my brain and body time to rest and reset?
- Am I having enough fun?
- Do I take time to care for my mental and physical health, or am I just focused on what I need to do?

See what you can change in your life to give yourself the time you need to rest. Watch something funny, spend time with a loved one, or do something that makes you smile. You can even schedule this into your day so you don't forget to take the time to enjoy life. Give yourself permission to slow down, rest, and fail. Remember that you are a human, not a robot!

You can use the following "help in a hurry" table to practice this in your life. You can also write it down in another way that works for you or download this table with spaces to work into using the QR code at the end of the chapter.

"I Feel Exhausted All the Time."	
Mindhack	Think about three things in your day that usually go underappreciated. These things can be objects, people, or events—it's up to you. The point of this exercise is to simply give thanks for the seemingly insignificant things in life. It is good to pause and just exist in the moment and appreciate what we do have instead of focusing on just what we need to do.
What am I thinking?	I am always tired! What is wrong with me? Why does life feel like it's too much?
How do I feel?	I am battling to sleep, and I feel guilty and nauseous every time I think about resting but then remember how much I still need to do.
Mindshift	I need to schedule more breaks and fun into my life so that I feel more rested and can actually do what I need to get done. I will do this by reading more novels, going for coffee with friends, and taking more walks in nature (or whatever I think will be restorative)!

7. How to Deal with "I Will Never Amount to Anything."

Take the time to observe and analyze your internal dialogue. Do you feel like you constantly put yourself down for not meeting your own expectations?

Of course, expectations are a normal part of life. We expect certain things from ourselves and others, and we also have to deal with the expectations of others in our life, whether at school, home, or work. However, too often these expectations become so burdensome that they lead to anxiety, panic attacks, burnout, and mental fatigue—especially when they are coming from deep inside us. It is amazing how easy it is to become our own worst critic!

The need to achieve at a certain level in front of others can come from a variety of factors, such as the perceived need to maintain a standard we have already achieved (like high grades) or the desire to not disappoint someone we look up to or care for. Athletes, speakers, CEOs, performing artists, managers, chefs, students, children, parents . . . we all experience the need to act in certain ways, which can often leave us feeling anxious about our own worth if we fail or make a mistake.

One of the main reasons we can experience self-imposed performance anxiety is due to the fact that we base our identity on a role we play. For instance, athletes often define their identity on their ability to perform a specific action on field—every time they play their sport, their identity is in a state of uncertainty, which can make them insecure and anxious about who they are and their self-worth, especially if they do not win. Yet there are a variety of factors involved in winning, and sometimes we just have bad days—this is often out of our control.

In many cases, when we have certain goals or standards we cannot live up to (whether from ourselves or others), we can feel like a fraud, even though no one can perform perfectly all the time. We are so focused on the goal that we forget to enjoy the process, which makes it difficult for us to change or adjust our expectations.

Indeed, when we fail to meet our high, self-imposed standards time and time again, it can make us feel like we are complete failures and that we never do anything important or of note. Consequently, we may end up expecting less and less of ourselves and feel like we should give up before we even try.

If this sounds like you, take the time to analyze your self-expectations. Are you putting undue pressure on yourself to perform to a certain standard? Why? Consciously observe and write down your critical self-talk and how often it's happening. What drives your desire to perform in a certain way? Is this something you want for yourself, or is it a goal you think you should achieve because other people have said so or defined success in this way?

Next, work on creating reconceptualized statements to counter this way of thinking and change the way you speak to yourself. For example, change "I wish I could be as good as . . ." to "I will never be able to live up to someone else's example of success because I am unique and I define my own success."

This will take time to become a habit, so make sure to practice it every day! The "help in a hurry" table just below is a great way to do this. You can also write it down in another way that works for you or download this table with spaces to work into using the QR code at the end of the chapter.

"I Will Never Amount to Anything."	
Mindhack	Listen to some favorite music that you know makes you feel good for a few minutes. Happy tunes can help lift your mood and help you feel better about yourself.
What am I thinking?	I will never amount to anything.
How do I feel?	I am so angry at myself that I feel sick. I get so upset that I can barely do what I need to do. I am so exhausted that I just want to crawl into a ball and hide forever. Everything feels so hopeless.
Mindshift	I will consciously and deliberately observe and write down my critical self-talk. Then I will think about what I am good at and what I have achieved. I will write this down to remind myself of what I can do and that I define my own success. I don't have to be good at everything! I am enough as I am.

Identifying and Tracking Which Pressures Affect You the Most

It's a really good idea to work out which of these seven pressures, or which combination of them, are putting the most pressure on you and disrupting your mental health. To help you do this, below is a simple process to follow and a table you can fill in whenever needed to help you organize your thinking. You can also write it down in another way that works for you or download this table with spaces to work into using the QR code at the end of the chapter.

The tracking process:

1. Observe yourself over the next week to find your "pressure cooker" signs.
2. Note in the table below each time you are affected by one of these pressures, what exactly you said/thought to put yourself under pressure, and how it made you feel.
3. Take note of how often this pops up in your life and what triggered it: who, what, when, where, and why.
4. After about one week of observing your thoughts, words, and behavior, take each sign you observed and work on it using the tips and "help in a hurry" tables above. If you are dealing with more than one, work on what is bothering you the most first.

Tracking Your "Pressure Cooker" Signs

The 7 "pressure cooker" signs	What I said/thought	Trigger (who, what, when, where, why—and how often)
I didn't get *x* done.		
I have to have it all together.		
I must succeed.		
I cannot make a mistake.		

(continued)

The 7 "pressure cooker" signs	What I said/thought	Trigger (who, what, when, where, why—and how often)
I will let everyone down.		
I feel exhausted all the time.		
I will never amount to anything.		

To download the tables from this chapter, visit helpinahurrybook.com/resources

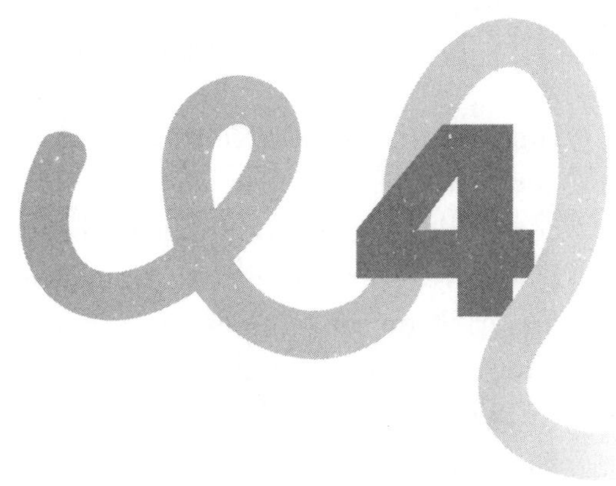

Help, My Brain Won't Shut Up!

Do you often find yourself overanalyzing every situation? Overthinking every conversation? Getting more and more upset the more you think about an experience or social interaction? Do you keep replaying scenarios in your head? Do you wish your brain would just shut up sometimes?

I think we can all relate to this on some level! It is normal to think about possible outcomes and scenarios and ask yourself questions about a past experience or even something you are currently going through. Here, it is important to differentiate between overthinking and deep thinking. Deep thinking is analyzing information for the purposes of learning and moving forward, building the brain, reaching solutions, and understanding difficult concepts.

Sometimes, this means we will need to think deeply about an issue we are facing in order to overcome it, but this is different from worrying about the problem. Deep thinking is really like what I like to call a "mental autopsy," where you reflect on and analyze your thoughts and feelings, adopting the role of a detective to identify patterns, triggers, and activators so you can change them. It's very deliberate, controlled, intentional, systematic, and rational. Say, for example, someone says something hurtful about you in anger. Deep thinking means you do not just react based on your feelings alone: Even though what was said was painful, you think about what was said, why the person may have said it, and how to best respond without escalating the situation. Your thoughts and actions are not emotionally driven, chaotic, illogical, assumptive, or led by a sense of victimization.

Deep thinking looks for a solution and closure, whereas overthinking is chaotic, with no solution or end in sight. For instance, using the example above, overthinking means you take what that person said in anger and marinate in it, thinking about it and letting your emotions overcome your logic and allowing what that person said to become part of you and define who you are.

Even though this sounds simple enough, it is also easy to fall into the overthinking trap, where we keep asking "what if" and ruminate on what should have happened, what could have happened, or what will happen, even though we know we cannot change the past or control how other people choose to react. One study from the University of Michigan shows 73 percent of adults ages twenty-five to thirty-five battle with negative rumination, while around 52 percent of those ages forty-five to fifty-five also struggle with overthinking.[1] So many of us battle with this, myself included.

But *why*? When we overthink something, we are essentially trying to process and understand it, especially if what has happened is out of the norm, hurtful, or painful. This is kind of like hearing an odd noise in the house while reading a book in bed—the sound is out of place and is, as a result, all the more jarring. These kinds of experiences go against our mind-brain-body network's natural optimism bias, which is designed to anticipate and hope for the best and helps balance our psychoneurobiology.[2]

Negative experiences are quite shocking because they throw us off balance, and our attention is drawn to restoring this balance. It is like our mind and brain are sending flashing red warning signals to us, telling us something happened and we need to figure it out before things get worse. We do this by thinking about the situation more to regain a sense of equilibrium through understanding and, hopefully, achieving some degree of closure.

It's easy for this process to spiral out of control, however, especially if we are in a more emotional and sensitive state or just more emotional and sensitive in general. Not that there's anything wrong with being very in touch with our feelings, but they can also be a launchpad into toxic rumination if not managed, which can make it feel like it is just us against a world that is out to get us.

Indeed, when it comes to overthinking, we have to be careful not to develop a victim mentality, where we keep ruminating over what has happened to us, staying stuck in the past without working on actually healing. Yes, people hurt us, and we hurt people, and bad things happen, but just overthinking a situation does not lead to closure. Closure requires deliberate and intentional mental work and time.

When we start overthinking a situation where we are to blame, there is a strong possibility we can end up trying to justify and reason away our behavior rather than using the situation to learn and grow. But when we try to make sense of a negative situation through blaming others rather than looking at ourselves, we cannot find true closure. The blame game is a never-ending toxic loop that forces us to overthink the words and actions of others. Taking responsibility for our choices and their impact, on the other hand, forces us to act and resolve a situation. Of course, even though the latter sounds better, it is more painful. Because who enjoys admitting they messed up? I know I certainly don't—but I also know I feel so much better when I do apologize and learn from my mistakes, even if it is initially quite uncomfortable to do so.

In many cases, overthinking is a result of the *assumptions* we make about another person's behavior, based on nonverbal cues like body language or tone, without getting clarification. The more we think about these assumptions and how they make us feel, the more it will influence our future words, behaviors, attitudes, and social interactions. We create a toxic cycle that holds us back from improving our social interactions and is often based on how we perceive something rather than what another person is actually thinking.

Two Signs to Watch Out For

Over extended periods of time, this kind of thinking will essentially create neural networks of anxiety in the mind-brain-body network, forming a bad habit that subjects our psychoneurobiology to long periods of stress and makes us more vulnerable to ill-health. This is why it is so important to be aware of and tuned in to how we are feeling and what we are thinking! It can have very real consequences on our well-being and keep us feeling trapped, stressed out, and overwhelmed.

When it comes to negative rumination and overthinking, there are two major signs to watch out for: the inability to focus and feelings of discomfort and anxiety.

The Inability to Focus

When you find your mind hopping from one thought to another and are unable to concentrate properly, this can be a sign you are stressed out from overthinking.

For example, say you have to deal with a difficult family member and are worried about what this person will say or do at your next gathering. You fret over this person's behavior for several days, are unable to focus at work or at home, and keep hopping from one imagined scenario to another. Soon, you feel sick from the stress, have an upset stomach every time you eat, and can't fall asleep at night because a thousand negative thoughts pop into your head as you switch off the light. Overthinking essentially taxes your ability to think deeply about any one thing, impeding your ability to examine and understand information.

Feelings of Discomfort and Anxiety

Overthinking can put your brain and body into negative stress, which can result in feelings of anxiety, depression, and fear and may even cause panic attacks. In fact, ruminating on negative thoughts is one of the biggest predictors of mental ill-health and is incredibly toxic for the brain and body, so it really is so important to become aware of what we think, how we feel, and how we choose to react.

If this resonates with you, remember: You are not alone! These are common thinking patterns we all tend to fall into at times that, thankfully, can be reversed and healed. Here are some "help in a hurry" tips you can use in the moment to help you catch yourself when you fall into the overthinking trap, manage your thinking, and reduce your stress levels.

1. Practice Deep Thinking

When we think deeply, we build our brain in a healthy way, increasing our cognitive resilience and mental flexibility, which improves how we deal with difficult situations. It involves the deliberate and intentional process of asking, answering, and discussing information to get meaning, develop understanding, and take action steps. This helps the brain develop and grow in a healthy way, taking advantage of the process of *neurogenesis*, or using the new baby nerve cells our brain creates on a daily basis to build new neural networks and form new behaviors.

A simple and easy way to practice this type of thinking is by reading. It harnesses the brain's ability to generate new ideas and envision new worlds, which is an aspect of deep thinking that activates neuroplasticity as it involves forming new neural connections and pathways in the mind-brain-body network.

Reading can also help calm down our neurophysiology enough for us to refocus and reduce the feelings of anxiety that go hand in hand with overthinking. Think of it as a really helpful distraction in the moment when we feel like our brain just will not shut off!

Reading is a fast and efficient way to turbo-boost the brain's ability to change and heal by helping generate healthy waves of balanced energy in the mind that sweep through the brain and body, supporting the immune and endocrine systems and the HPA (hypothalamic-pituitary-adrenal) axis, which can help us better deal with stress and negative circumstances.

The deep thinking that comes from reading can also result in changes in gamma, alpha, beta, delta, and theta brain waves, which are associated with learning, an optimal state of relaxation and alertness, and bridging between the conscious and nonconscious mind, all of which can help support peacefulness, readiness, creativity, and meditation—pretty useful habits that can help us counter overthinking and negative rumination in the moment.

To start practicing this in your life, set aside some time and find a great book, fiction or nonfiction, and schedule in a specific amount of time to read. I recommend starting with thirty minutes to an hour. You can even read the news, an article, or whatever interests you! The key is to find something that engages you so you are not easily distracted.

2. Ask Questions

If you find yourself overthinking a situation or problem that involves another person, take the time to ask them for more clarification before making assumptions. Ask them what they mean and why they said what they said or did what they did. This will help avoid the misunderstandings and overthinking that come as a result of miscommunication.

But be sure to calm down before angrily or reactively snapping back. A great way to do this is by applying what I call the ten-second rule. Pause for ten seconds to breathe deeply, in and out. I have found that the easiest way to do this is to breathe in for three seconds, then out for seven seconds. You can repeat this as many times as necessary, which will help calm down your mind and brain, improve your decision-making, and reduce impulsivity. Once you feel more in control, you can then respond to the situation instead of just allowing yourself to fall into an overthinking spiral based solely on conjectures.

3. Schedule a Time to Worry, Then Take Action

This may sound odd, but scheduling a time to worry or think about something and then making an action plan can be incredibly helpful. Limiting the amount of time you spend thinking about the problem with a timer or stopwatch can help you avoid endlessly ruminating on the issue and experiencing emotional burnout, mental fatigue, and increased anxiety, while having an action plan for what to do after this time has ended will help you feel like you are achieving some sense of closure. Action plans can include forgiving the person, setting a new boundary to improve the relationship, or apologizing and finding a way to make amends that shows you truly mean what you say, depending on the situation you find yourself in. And you don't need to do this for long; literally a couple of minutes, as needed, does the trick!

4. Think About What You Can Learn from the Situation

Rather than just worrying about a particular situation, think about how you can learn from it. Take a few minutes to consider the situation, asking yourself why it happened like it did, talking about it out loud with yourself or a loved one, and thinking about how you can improve the situation to get the outcome you desire.

What does closure look like for you? How do you want this situation to play out? Ask yourself a lot of deliberate questions to help direct your thinking, rather than just let your mind run ahead of you. This objective self-questioning helps restore a sense of autonomy over the situation and also disrupts the mind-brain-body network from settling into a negative habit.

5. Pretend You Are Advising a Friend or Loved One

Imagine your friend or loved one is experiencing what you are going through and has come to you for help. This will help you objectify the issue, almost as if you are standing outside of yourself and looking in, which, in turn, will help you calm down the overthinking reaction you are experiencing and come up with a way to move forward.

To practice this, ask yourself these three questions and answer with a few simple sentences in as clinical and objective a way as possible, as though you are talking your loved one through this issue.

1. *What are you thinking right now, and why?*

   Example: I shared too much the last time I spoke to this person, so they probably want nothing to do with me. They are going to tell everyone about me, and other people will think that there is something wrong with me.
2. *How does this make you feel?*

   Example: I feel nauseous, and I have a terrible headache. I can't concentrate, and I feel really sad and hopeless. I can't stop thinking about what happened and why.
3. *What can you do to quit this overthinking spiral and move forward?*

   Example: This person may not like me, or I may be making an assumption that is false. I do not know what they are thinking, and my fears are based on my own perceptions about myself rather than what they said. I can speak to this person once I have calmed down, but I also recognize that in order to heal I need to work on how I see myself and how I talk to myself, or I will always assume people are talking about me or think I am overwhelming.

Here is a simple table you can use to work through these three questions, or you can write it down in another way that works for you or download it using the QR code at the end of the chapter.

Three Questions to Stop Overthinking

Question	Answer
1. What are you thinking right now?	
2. How does this make you feel?	
3. What can you say/think to get yourself out of this overthinking spiral and move forward?	

And finally, here is a list of some phrases to help you with the "moving forward" part of this exercise, which is the hardest step.

To Move Forward

Type of overthinking	**What can you say/think to get yourself out of this overthinking spiral and move forward?**
You find yourself going down the path of "This will happen."	The chance of "this" actually happening is very low. Why waste energy worrying about "what if" when you can use this energy to learn what you can, move on, and focus on making your next moment your best moment?
You feel like you keep trying and failing, so why bother?	Every time you try, you are learning something new and expanding your intelligence and resilience. Every time you fail, you are learning what *not* to do next time! So, what did you learn this time?
There are so many options—what do you do?	Count your options. Now, reduce them to the top three, then top two, then follow through on the one that's left.
This person is going to do this or say that.	You don't know what they are thinking or what they will do, so don't waste your mental energy going down this road. Rather, focus on what your assumptions are telling you about yourself and what you need to work on, and make the time to ask that person what they meant or what they are thinking, rather than just assuming you know.
You wish you could go back and redo the past.	You can't change or undo the past. You can only change how you see the situation and how you respond to it. So, what are you going to do?
You feel like you don't understand what happened and are drowning in all the details of the experience.	Look at the big picture. What would someone else say about this situation? Can you work on accepting the unacceptable? How will the issues floating around in your mind affect you tomorrow, in six months, in a year, or in five years?
You feel like you need a break from your own head.	The quickest way to get out of your own head is to do something nice for someone else. So, what are you going to do? How can you help someone in your life? How can you make someone else's day better?

(continued)

Type of overthinking	What can you say/think to get yourself out of this overthinking spiral and move forward?
You feel like you always mess up.	Write down three to five things you succeeded at doing in the last day or two, or think of something you've achieved that you are proud of. Do you really feel like you always do the wrong thing? Do you give yourself permission to make mistakes? You are only human, after all!
You feel like no one likes you.	Why do you feel this way? Can you see what was said or done from a different perspective? Did you perhaps do something wrong? Making a mistake does not make you a bad person. Do you feel this way when you mess up?
You can't stop thinking about what happened.	Choose to spend a specific amount of time (e.g., five to ten minutes) thinking about what has passed, then choose to forgive, apologize, or whatever is appropriate to the situation you find yourself in. If you spend too much time ruminating on the problem, you will get caught up in the emotions associated with the toxic thinking pattern, which can lead to emotional burnout, mental fatigue, and increased anxiety. It is best to spend a limited amount of time defining what the issue is and focus more on what you can do to improve the situation. So, what is your plan of action?

To download the tables from this chapter, visit helpinahurrybook.com/resources

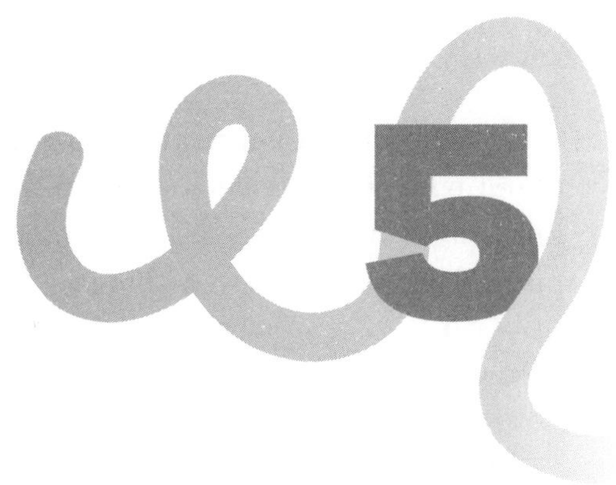

Help, I Want to Punch That Person in the Face!

Let's face it: People can be irritating. Indeed, things can get so toxic that a deserted cabin in the middle of the wilderness can sound quite appealing, especially if you *have* just punched that person in the face . . .

Unfortunately, resorting to violence is not great for our mental health or relationships, and we cannot just run away from everyone who annoys us. Every day, we can potentially face a negative social interaction, whether via an email, text message, conversation, meeting, gathering, or similar. We need to learn how to deal with such situations, not run from them (or punch anyone in the face).

Yes, toxic people can be upsetting and can mess with our emotions and mental health. But this means that the sooner we learn to manage our reactions to the way other people treat us, the better off we will be (both mentally and physically).

This is not just necessary for people we don't like or get along with. Even friends and family can, unknowingly or knowingly, create stressful environments. I once read a quote online that really stuck with me:

> You will continue to suffer if you have an emotional reaction to everything that is said to you. True power is observing things with logic. True power is restraint. If words control you that means everyone else can control you. Breathe and allow things to pass.[1]

Though I can't say where this quote originally came from, it has helped me so much that I wanted to share it with you and also give you some "help in a hurry" tips that have really helped me and others learn how to manage toxic people in the moment when things really feel like they are spiraling out of control.

The key thing to remember is that you can't control what another person chooses to think, say, or do, but you *can* control your reactions to them! If you choose to give people power over you by continually ruminating over what they said or did and reacting to them, you will continue to suffer, negatively impacting your mind, brain, body, and mental health in the process and compounding the toxic effects that person has on you.

This is especially the case if you have developed a pattern of overreacting to that person; you can get stuck in a toxic reaction cycle that will further affect the quality of your mental life. If this sounds familiar, it's a good idea to stop from time to time and ask yourself, *What kind of person am I becoming?* Do you want to keep suffering like this? Are you developing a victim mentality? Does it feel like it is always you against the world?

In many cases, when it comes to dealing with toxic people, true power is restraint. It is key in helping us manage toxic situations, as when we do not develop our self-restraint and self-regulation, we can make ourselves pretty miserable!

This starts with our thought life. It is important to remember that you can never truly know someone else's thoughts or motivations, even if you know the person well, and assumptions are, by and large, the origin of a lot of mess-ups!

At the end of the day, we will never truly know what motivates someone's words or actions. We may be able to guess to a certain extent, but we will never get beyond a 70 percent accuracy rate, so we need to stop ourselves from going down that dangerous road. Assumptions are often toxic; we can end up wasting a lot of our mental energy on things that do not contribute to our quality of life or our success.

Restraint also means taking the time to step back and observe a situation logically. This means reminding yourself that, in many social situations, you have control—you aren't under someone's power unless *you allow it*. There are always exceptions, including extreme cases of abuse (which is beyond the purview of this book), but for the average social interaction, you have power over how you choose to respond to the other person.

The reality is, if you let your toxic emotions toward someone grow unchecked by constantly thinking about them and ruminating on how they have hurt you and what they have done and what they will do, you will feel worse. The resultant neurochemical chaos can make you more vulnerable to mental and physical ill-health. Do you really want to give people that much power over your life? Remember, if words control you, then everyone can control you! Punching someone in the face, metaphorically or otherwise, may feel good in the moment, but it can have some serious repercussions in your life. Short-term gain, long-term pain, as the saying goes.

It is so important that we control how we react and respond to people, not just for the sake of our relationships but also for our mental health. We should not let people walk all over us, but we should not let our emotions walk all over us either! It is possible to be firm and defend ourselves, mitigate relationship disasters, and improve our own mental health.

This does not mean we all need to agree on everything. Rather, it is about embracing the old adage that it is often okay to agree to disagree, and sometimes we don't know everything!

If you are constantly falling prey to what other people do or say, you need to be honest with yourself: Are you letting your emotions and other people control you? Do you want this to be your life? If not, you need to work on managing how you feel and react in the moment, which, over time and with practice, can become a habit. Here are some "help in a hurry" tips to help you do this when you really want to slap that person in the face.

1. Practice Deep Breathing

This may sound simple or useless, but so many of us don't really think about our breathing or how powerful a tool it can be when it comes to our mental health. Breathing in and out deeply can help us learn how to control our cortisol and adrenaline levels, which, if left unchecked, can cause havoc when they flood the brain and body. It can also help calm the HPA axis, which helps us feel less reactive and more in control in the moment.

Oxygen also carries information.[2] When we breathe really deeply and slowly, we are sucking in large volumes of "information," which is telling our brain and body that things are okay, and this lowers our physiological arousal. This, in turn, will help us get more clarity of thought and defog our mind.

For example, say you were just sent a nasty email from a colleague. Instead of responding in a reactive way, stop and breathe in and out super deeply. This will dissipate excess cortisol and help your mind clear and your emotions stabilize, giving that person less control over you in the moment and protecting your well-being!

Some great ways to practice deep breathing are:

- *Box breathing*: Inhale through your nose for four seconds, hold your breath for four seconds, exhale from your mouth for four seconds, and then hold your breath for four seconds. Repeat this as many times as necessary. Focus on how your breath feels going in and out or how this type of breathing is calming down your mind and brain. You can even visualize what you think this looks like in your brain and support this with a statement like, "I can have a moment before I respond."
- *Ten-second pause breathing*: Breathe in for around three counts and breathe out for around seven counts. If you want, you can put your hand on your stomach and feel it rise up in the inhalation; on the exhalation, you can "whoosh" it out forcefully, which pushes oxygen to the front of the brain. Repeat this around six to nine times, for sixty to ninety seconds—or for however long you can manage.
- *Use your nose*: Using gentle finger pressure to block the other nostril, breathe in through one side of your

nose and out the other side, which can also help you decompress.

2. Visualize, Visualize, Visualize!

Here are three great visualization exercises you can do quickly alongside or instead of deep breathing. They literally take a few seconds. You can do one, two, or all three—whatever you need in the moment! These exercises will give you some temporary relief and help calm down your heart rate and cortisol levels so that you can respond better to a negative person.

- *A box in the sea*: As you are listening to the person who is triggering you, visualize putting that person inside a box, closing the lid, and throwing it far out to sea. See it floating away to a place where the person can't bother you.
- *Shrinking people*: As you look at the person who is affecting you, imagine them shrinking into tiny, tiny versions of themselves, so tiny you can't even see them or hear what they are saying.
- *Wearing armor*: Visualize yourself in a coat of armor. See this in your mind's eye protecting you from the "arrows" the other person is shooting at you. This armor is so strong that all those "barbs" are just bouncing off you into the air. As you do this, it will generate positive energy in your mind and brain, which acts like a shield that will help you divorce your own emotions from the situation and give your mind a break from the stress. It is also a great way to remind yourself that you are strong and protected

from the negative side effects of the person's words and actions so that you don't react impulsively toward them.

3. Recognize and Name Your Reaction

Don't ignore how you feel! Acknowledge it, validate it—then work on moving on rather than letting your emotions take over and control you. For instance, using the email example above, describe how you feel out loud: "I feel hurt, attacked, defensive . . ." and ask yourself *why*.

Writing down your thoughts and feelings can help you manage them better. The simple act of putting them down on paper or on your phone or device creates some distance from how you feel, allowing you to calm down instead of responding in a reactive way. You are getting them out instead of keeping them in.

But don't do this for too long, just for a few moments! You don't want to ruminate on your feelings. The purpose of this exercise is to help you name and describe your reactions. Writing can help bring fluency and clarity to your thinking and reduce the overwhelming effect of the negative energy generated by toxic people.

4. Have a Discussion with Yourself and Come Up with an Action Plan

This tip works really well with the ones above or on its own. You can also have your discussion with a mental health professional or loved one if you feel like you need additional help or perspective on this issue.

Intentionally and deliberately separate your emotions from the logic of the situation. Visualize a dark tree that is formed from all of your reactions. Imagine stripping the emotions off this tree, as if you are picking off all the leaves. Now you can see the well-defined branches with all the information of the situation hanging on the tree in a clear and clinical way, which will give you insight into what to do next. You are essentially imagining taking the threat of the turbulent emotions away from your thought "tree."

Now, focus on the content and words of this tree, which will help you see the actual problem or issue for what it is. Trying to see things through a veil of emotion is like trying to drive through a storm with no windshield wipers—you can't always see properly and can end up in some serious trouble!

When you mentally divorce yourself from your immediate emotional reaction, you can often see things more clearly and come up with an action plan. For example, by noting that the person who sent the email is frustrated because of "so and so," you can put yourself in their shoes and *choose* to see if there is something you can learn from the situation in order to improve your communication with this person rather than letting your emotions dominate you in the moment. By doing this, you can transform a potentially explosive situation into a productive learning experience.

We need to validate how we feel, yes, but we can't just focus on our feelings; they are only one part of the bigger picture. When we have created distance between what happened and what we feel about it, we can then work on a plan of action: finding concrete solutions to move forward and use the situation to learn and grow.

Here are two examples of what this could look like:

My Action Plan

Toxic statement/situation that upset me	
I had a discussion with someone who blames me for saying something that put them in a bad light.	I received a toxic email from someone at work.
How do I feel about this?	
I feel frustrated and hurt because I didn't have to say anything to anyone; their own actions did all the talking.	I feel shocked and thrown off. I was not expecting this email or the way this person is attacking me.
Answer and discuss with myself	
I know the truth. I also think I know why this person is saying this—they are struggling. However, I need to talk to someone about how to handle this because it's happening so much that I feel emotionally abused. Maybe there is a better way I can handle this in the future, and talking to someone I trust will help me get a different perspective and help me better manage this situation.	I am going to try to mentally separate myself from my immediate emotional reaction. Okay, so knowing what I do about this person, perhaps they are frustrated because of "so and so," and, putting myself in their shoes, I can see why they responded the way they did and why they think I am to blame. However, even though they are wrong and their response was toxic, I am going to choose to learn from the situation in order to improve my communication with this person. I will say x and see if I can help them process this in a healthier way. I will respond in a composed and logical manner to my colleague and set up a call or in-person meeting to calmly discuss the situation and improve our future communication, because things are often lost in translation over email.

To download the table from this chapter, visit helpinahurrybook .com/resources

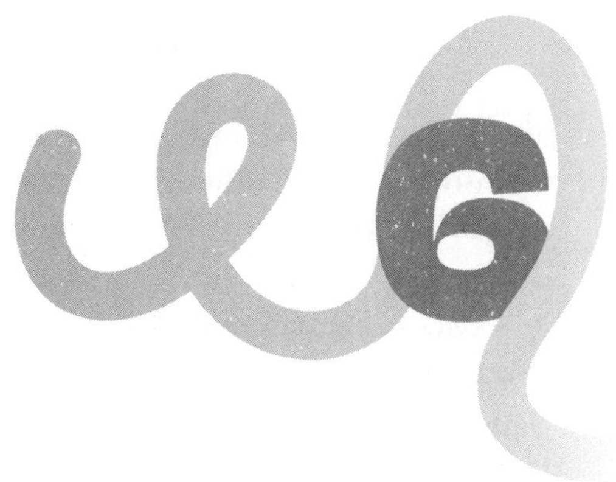

Help, the World Seems So Black-and-White!

Have you ever caught yourself thinking that there is only a right or wrong way to think, with no in-between? This is called black-and-white thinking, and even though it's pretty common, it can make us feel frustrated and stuck. Life exists on a spectrum, which means that sometimes we have to embrace the gray areas or we will quickly find ourselves trapped in our own cognitive distortions.

Another way to understand black-and-white thinking is as "all-or-nothing" thinking.[1] Being human is not simple, so neither should be the way we think about and approach life. Many things have many causes, and in some cases, right or wrong comes face-to-face with moral ambiguity. Some conflicts exist without good or bad sides, and some problems have no right answers. All-or-nothing thinking tends to overlook this, keeping us trapped in an "either/or" mindset that can leave us upset, anxious, or angry.

This is why it is so important we learn to embrace "gray" or "both/and" thinking to deal with the hard challenges of the real world. We need to step away from seeing the world in extremes and absolutes and acknowledge that much of life exists in the realm of "sometimes/maybe" rather than "always/never."

Indeed, if we are unable to see alternatives in a situation or possible solutions to a problem, we can end up negatively impacting our mental health and life. We may end up punishing ourselves if we do not do something exactly "right" or fail to meet our own high standards, or we may end up overlooking how important we are to others. With black-and-white thinking, we can quickly become hopeless or depressed and feel like we have little to no worth.

Take the extremely common adage "No pain, no gain." This is such a great example of black-and-white thinking. Sure, in many situations pain is required to "gain," when we are talking about the struggle of learning something new, working out, changing a habit, or even healing trauma. But this is just one perspective, and it leaves a lot unsaid. As author and longevity expert Dan Buettner notes, the opposite is also true: When there's no pain, there's gain—because when there's no pain, you're more likely to do it every day![2]

Reality is a lot more complicated than simple adages convey, and I think this is something many of us intrinsically know but find hard to comprehend when things feel like they are falling apart around us. The black-and-white statements we use or ideas we have can easily obscure just how uncertain and complicated life can truly be. They can make us feel guilty when we don't feel like our thoughts fit what we are experiencing, or they can even make us feel like we are "doing life wrong" when things change or when we experience the unknown, which can have a real strain on our mental health and relationships.

Life is not an "either/or" game. It is a "both/and" game, which means it is *normal* to hold two or more opposing ideas or feelings at the same time, and accepting this will save us a lot of mental distress. For example, you can love someone but need to pull back a bit so you aren't enabling them or supporting toxic behaviors that harm them. Or there may be someone in your life whom you love very much, but something they are doing is triggering what you are working on in your own life, so you need to temporarily create some space or set up some boundaries for yourself. It is not unusual that someone may be toxic for you right now, where you are at. This doesn't mean it's a permanent thing, nor does it mean you are a bad person.

It's completely normal for situations and relationships to change over time or for things to feel uncertain. Indeed, we literally rewire our brain at each stage in life with our mind, which is why shifts in relationships and situations take some getting used to and can feel strange at first. It doesn't mean things are "wrong."

If you feel like you often succumb to a black-and-white way of thinking and it is impacting how you experience and manage life, the most important thing you can do is take the time to observe yourself and note down how you are thinking about situations and how you talk to yourself. Notice what patterns you can observe in your own life, what your triggers are, and how you can work on changing your responses and way of thinking in the moment when you are battling to see the gray in your world. The tips below are designed to help you practice this in your life!

However, as I've mentioned in previous chapters, if you recognize this as a pattern in your life, it's also important to make small changes over at least 63 days to change the mind-brain-body network and develop a sustainable habit, which I discuss in detail in my other books and my app, Neurocycle.

1. Move Away from Absolutes

Observe yourself over a couple of days to see if and how often you are using absolute words such as *always*, *never*, and *ever*. Then, think about why you use those words and what you can use as alternatives to help shift your perspective from black-and-white thinking to seeing and accepting life's more complicated gray areas.

Below is a list of absolute words and phrases with space for you to tally how often you use each one over a period of three to seven days, as well as a space to come up with alternative words. I have added some of the most common ones, but you are welcome to change these or add more.

You can also create your own table or download one by using the QR code at the end of the chapter—whatever works best for you! As mentioned, you can add more words as you see fit or change any of the titles/phrases based on your own experiences, which is why there are several blank spaces at the bottom of the table.

Absolutes and Alternatives

Absolute word/phrase	How often	When, where	Alternative
Always			Sometimes Usually Frequently With some exceptions

Absolute word/phrase	How often	When, where	Alternative
Never			Maybe Sometimes Rarely Hardly any Infrequently
Ever			Now and then
None			A few Little Rare Hardly any
Must Should			Maybe I could I would like to I can I may
Everyone Everybody			A lot of people Some people Many people

(continued)

Absolute word/phrase	How often	When, where	Alternative
Nobody No one			A small number of people One or two people Only a few people
I need to be all in			I can only try my best.
No pain, no gain			This isn't necessarily true; hard work doesn't always involve pain but it does take perseverance, and I have that in me.
Bragging rights start at 60 hours per week			I love my work, and whether I work 10 or 60 hours a week, I am proud of what I do, but my worth is not based on how much I work. There is value in rest.
You either succeed or fail in life			Success may not look like how I expect. My failures teach me a lot about life and help me succeed. Life is not just about succeeding at something. I define my own success.

2. Develop a Mindset That Seeks Alternatives and Generates Possibilities

Working on changing your mindset is a great way to quit black-and-white thinking and practice tapping into your unlimited resilience reserves so it becomes a habit when you need it most, which is when life feels unknown and uncertain.

A mindset is a way your mind functions, like a habit. It is a way you "set" your mind, literally. Like planting your garden in the spring yields amazing results all year if you do it right, deliberately choosing and practicing a mindset can really help you when life hits hard. That is why I often call mindsets "insurance policies"—they are there for you when you need them the most.

Practicing a mindset that seeks alternatives and generates possibilities is incredibly helpful when it comes to quitting the trap of black-and-white thinking. This kind of mindset looks for different ways of arriving at a judgment, understanding a situation, or solving a problem. It allows you to embrace life's uncertainties and manage how you feel when you enter those gray areas that are an intrinsic part of life.

A great way to do this is to make the decision to try, as much as possible, to look for three to five possibilities before deciding on one in any given situation. This gives you the chance to come up with something different, and maybe even better, than the black-and-white option. Even if you find yourself coming back to that option, the mere consideration of alternatives enables you to tap into your creativity, expanding your perspective and helping you look beyond the black-and-white.

For example, think of a time when you felt like a failure: You didn't do something right, which means you did something wrong. Right? Not necessarily! On the one hand, you didn't do something as it was supposed to be done. Technically, you were "wrong." But this is wrong with a lowercase *w*. On the other hand, then, this experience taught you something and helped you grow. This is another way to look at the situation and see it as a possibility to help you succeed later on in life.

Training your mind to think in this way will help develop your intelligence and insight, making you more resilient to the ups and downs of life. It teaches you how to dig deep into the wisdom of your nonconscious mind (which I spoke about in chapter 2) and find solutions and ways through the challenges you face. It is a mindset that is characterized by perseverance and hope, even when things feel uncertain or weird!

Indeed, the more you practice this mindset, the more you will find yourself applying it to many different areas in your life. If one door closes, you will start seeing another one open. For example, maybe you are in a reorganizational phase in your business; imagining four to five (or more!) different possibilities and writing them down helps you see things from a different perspective and really figure out what you want to do and why. And when you go into the actual process of strategizing, you'll already have a springboard to start from, even if one strategy doesn't work out. You are more resilient to change, which is one of the best skills you can develop as you go through life!

Below is a simple table you can use to start practicing this. You can also write it down in another way that works for you or download this table with spaces to work into using the QR code at the end of the chapter.

Possibilities and Alternatives

Situation:

Black-and-white view:

Alternative 1:

Alternative 2:

Alternative 3:

Alternative 4:

Alternative 5:

To download the tables from this chapter, visit helpinahurrybook .com/resources

To download the Neurocycle app, visit www.neurocycle.app

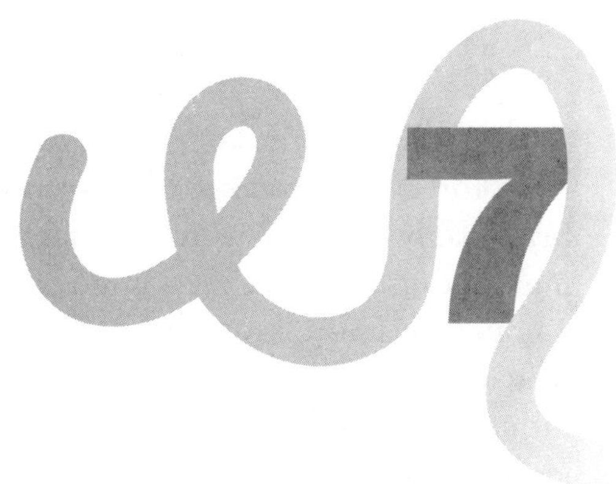

Help, I'm Tired All the Time!

How often does someone ask you how you are doing, and you say "I'm tired"? This is such a common response that we don't pay it much attention. What's new? We are *all* tired *all* the time.

But really, this is something we should be focusing on. It should come with flashing lights saying "Warning, warning, danger ahead!" Rest is an important part of maintaining a healthy mind, brain, and body, and it allows us to better respond to the challenges of life.

Without rest, we cannot function very well at all. Yes, our nonconscious mind never stops. It's always trying to make us aware of issues that are damaging our resilience and causing neurophysiological disruptions in our brain and body. However, the conscious mind and brain *do* get tired because they work on limited energy. Remember, this is kind of like when we have a whole lot of apps open on our phone, with the brightness on full, and we are constantly using it—very soon the battery will die.

Why? As we go through our day, everything we experience is captured and processed by our nonconscious mind and brain, only parts of which are filtered into the conscious mind because our conscious mind can only handle very small amounts of information at a time. During each day, a lot of neuroplasticity (brain change) is occurring—we will build around eight thousand new memories in thought clusters (neural networks) into our brain and body.[1] This activity drains our "battery," making our brain, conscious mind, and body tired because they have limited energy.

The conscious mind and brain can get tired even if we have a lot of good stuff happening in our life. This is often why, even when things are going well, we can feel a loss of drive and creativity and maybe even feel a little down.

So, like we need to recharge our phone, we also need to recharge our brain and conscious mind. It's best we do this in a regular way by incorporating periods of rest into our daily schedule to keep the brain charged all day long. Even a minute or two every hour, plus a fifteen-minute break every three hours, where we just switch off to the external and on to the internal can help so much to rest and regenerate ourselves. If we go for too long without rest, we may think we are okay, but the next day we won't feel as rested as we should. We may notice our ability to think clearly and respond to the ups and downs of life is off because we didn't recharge regularly and pushed our conscious mind and brain to the limit, again.

But resting is easier said than done. We all know, on some level, that we need it. We may even make a conscious effort to incorporate more periods of rest into our life, but we end up feeling just as exhausted and burned out as before. How many of us have ever binge-watched a Netflix show because we desperately needed a break, only to feel completely unrested the minute the binge ended? Or we take that weekend break or holiday but come back feeling like we are still exhausted, even though we spent hours lying on a beach and going for long walks in beautiful scenery?

If this is you, you are not alone! Every time I push beyond an eight-hour day thinking I will be okay, I feel a drop in my creativity and my mood the next day. Finding ways to truly rest and "switch off" can be incredibly challenging. Although there is a ton of information out there (just look at how many social media posts are encouraging you to make self-care a routine part of your regimen!), so many of us are still exhausted and burned out. It seems like almost every day there is a new article telling us how bad things are, but, for many of us, we don't even need to read it. We know firsthand how bad things are and how burned out we feel, and we are immersed in this message to the point where we spend more time thinking about how burned out we are than resting!

An important distinction to make when it comes to resting is the difference between simply giving our mind, brain, and body a chance to rest and truly taking the time to restore and reboot our psychoneurobiology.

Restoring is a transitive verb. It means to give back, to return, to put or bring back into existence and use . . . to renew. The opposite of restoration is to weaken, undermine, cripple, undo, depress, split, or dull. *Rest*, on the other hand, is defined as ceasing activity to relax and refresh, or to recover strength.[2]

We may get the "rest" bit right, but we often miss the "restore" element. So, for example, when we binge-watched that Netflix show or went to that exercise class or had fun with family and friends on that vacation, we may have been resting, but we were not necessarily giving our mind, brain, and body a chance to truly *restore*. Deep down, we may still have been worrying about that family member, that work we still had to do, how this person was going to react to that person, and so on. Instead of allowing our mind and brain to renew and restore and return to baseline, we were instead weakening, undermining, and undoing our rest, setting ourselves up for failure in the future.

Some signs that this may be happening in your life are:

- *Emotional changes*: You might feel gloomier, depressed, anxious, stuck in the past, and unable to enjoy things you used to love.
- *Brain fog*: You have more memory issues and cannot function mentally as well as you used to.
- *Relationship struggles*: You may notice you are more irritable and cranky and are taking this out on your loved ones, which is impacting your ability to truly connect with others and making you feel more alone.
- *Physical ill-health*: You may notice you're having more health issues like gastrointestinal discomfort or low energy, or maybe you're getting sick more often than you used to.

So, what can you do? Although this may sound counterintuitive, rest has so much to do with the mind—in fact, pretty much everything to do with the mind. Regardless of what technique we use or what things we do to rest, if we can't manage what is going through our mind, it can backfire on us, leaving us feeling tired, burned out, and unable to handle the challenges life throws our way.

Here are some quick and simple tips to help you manage your mind in the moment to rest *and* restore.

1. Take More Thinker Moments

Research shows that we spend half to three-quarters of our day in our mind time-traveling through our thoughts and memories. How we do this can either help or harm our ability to rest well, which is why it is important to take what I call "thinker moments" throughout the day.

Thinker moments are periods where we sort of "zone out," allowing our mind to switch from active problem-solving to wandering and daydreaming, which help us rest our conscious mind and physical brain. They give our brain the downtime needed to recharge and function optimally. When we let our mind wander, we internally reboot our thinking, giving our internal dialogue some quality "me time."

I have found that the best way to have a thinker moment is to close my eyes and allow my mind to release a free flow of thoughts for one to five minutes. Having a pen and paper (or phone/device) at hand is useful during this process so you can write down the thoughts that are flowing freely and their direction, as well as the thoughts you keep coming back to that are stealing your peace, which you can then work through at another time.

Another fun way to practice thinker moments is to read a novel or story for a bit, close your eyes, and let your mind just think about and "play around" with what you just read. It is a fast and efficient way of turbo-boosting the brain's ability to rest, change, and heal because it helps generate healthy waves of balanced energy in the mind, which then sweep through the brain and body, supporting the immune and endocrine systems and the HPA axis that can help you better deal with stress and negative circumstances. It can also result in changes in gamma, alpha, beta, delta, and theta brain waves, which are associated with learning, an optimal state of relaxation and alertness, and bridging between the conscious and nonconscious mind. These changes can help support peacefulness, readiness, creativity, and meditation.

These intermittent periods of mind-wandering are also critical for restoring our memory and creativity. It is one major reason why solutions and creative ideas, or "aha!" moments, often come unexpectedly during periods of rest or downtime. So, if you feel like you are in a slump mentally, practicing these thinker moments can also be really helpful.

2. Avoid "Milkshake" Multitasking

Even though we all tend to do it at times, multitasking is just not that great for the brain. Our conscious mind isn't good at this kind of scattered, jumpy thinking. It draws energy from our brain and creates something akin to a dust storm in our conscious mind, which can affect our rest, thereby impacting our mental and physical health.

When we multitask, we end up with what I call "milkshake thinking," which is the opposite of mindfulness. Every rapid, incomplete, and low-quality shift of thought makes a "milkshake" with our brain cells and neurochemicals and stresses out all the systems in our body, which is the opposite of how the brain is designed to function. When we consciously try to jump rapidly from one task to another, we essentially cloud our ability to concentrate and think deeply, which impacts our ability to do a task well, leading to unnecessary levels of anxiety and stress.

If you are anything like me, sometimes it is hard to resist the temptation to multitask, especially when you are resting. However, I've realized that when I consciously make an effort *not* to multitask, I really do feel more restored and renewed.

You can practice doing this in your life by choosing to deliberately and consciously focus on the present moment. Some people love focusing on their breathing to do this, imagining the air whooshing in and out of their lungs in the present moment. This simple exercise can be really helpful because it is easy to remember, especially when you are feeling overwhelmed. Focused breathing gets you "out of your brain" by keeping it busy with the technical aspects of breathing, allowing your more spiritual mind to dominate and to calm and focus you.

To do this, close your eyes and take a few slow, deep breaths. Inhale deeply through your nose, allowing your abdomen to expand, and exhale slowly through your mouth, letting go of any tension or stress with each breath. Bring your attention inward, focusing on the sensations within your body. Notice the gentle rise and fall of your chest as you breathe, the feeling of being grounded to the floor (or bed, if you're lying down), and how your body feels.

With each inhale, imagine drawing in calmness, peace, and clarity. Let these qualities fill your entire being, from the top of your head to the tips of your toes. As you exhale, imagine releasing any worries, doubts, or negative thoughts that may be weighing on your mind. Allow them to dissolve and drift away with each exhale. Take a moment to check in with yourself emotionally. Without judgment, notice any feelings or sensations that arise, simply allowing them to be present.

Continue to breathe deeply and mindfully, staying present with your inner experience. If your mind starts to wander, gently guide your focus back to your breath and the sensations within your body. Spend a few more moments in this state of inward reflection, savoring the stillness and quietude. What also helps with this is to do a few breaths where you say "Let" as you breathe in and "Go" as you breathe out.

Another helpful way to practice focusing on one thing in the moment instead of multitasking is this simple grounding exercise: acknowledging what is around you with your senses. Begin by finding a comfortable seated position and taking a few deep breaths in, allowing your body to relax with each exhale. First, take a moment to acknowledge five things you see around you. Notice the colors, shapes, and textures of each object.

Next, acknowledge four things you can touch around you. Feel the texture of the surface beneath you, the fabric of your clothing, or any other objects within reach.

Now shift your focus to three things you can hear. Perhaps close your eyes. Listen closely to the sounds around you, whether it's the hum of appliances, the rustle of leaves outside, or the gentle flow of your breathing.

Take another deep breath in and notice two things you can smell. Perhaps it's the aroma of a nearby candle, the scent of fresh air, or even the fragrance on your clothes.

Lastly, bring your awareness to one thing you can taste. It might be the lingering flavor of your last meal or a sip of water you just took. As you continue to take a few more deep breaths, allow yourself to fully immerse in the present moment, feeling grounded and centered in your surroundings. Savor the sensations of calm and tranquility flowing through you.

3. Make Your Rest Periods About Yourself, Not Other People

We need to make our rest periods about *our rest* and stop letting other people pull on our energy reserves when we are trying to restore our mind, brain, and body. Indeed, we can't truly help someone else or deal with them if they are on our mind all the time, because it will wear us down. I call this the "oxygen mask principle"—like in a plane, we have to put on our own oxygen mask before we can help others.

This means being careful about who we choose to surround ourselves with when we rest. Being around negative people can be incredibly draining. We need to balance our time with healthy people and healthy, happy conversations, enforce our personal boundaries when necessary, and also just be alone with our thoughts.

So, if you feel like you are not resting well, take a look at who you choose to surround yourself with when you are trying to take a break. Are they supporting or hurting your mental health? If the latter, what boundaries can you put in place to rest better? If you need some alone time, don't feel guilty! Saying no to someone or something is perfectly okay if this is what you need to rest. In fact, saying no to people who are self-centered, draining, or codependent is often necessary for our mental well-being. You can still be there for someone if they are in dire need, but you do not have to let them affect your ability to rest and restore.

4. Recognize That Restorative Rest Is Customizable, Not Prescriptive

When it comes to rest, don't pigeonhole yourself. Real, restorative rest is freeing, meaningful, and *customizable*. We are all different, and what may be restful for one person may be stressful for another. You need to find what works best for you and avoid trying to compare your needs to what other people are saying or doing.

Your version of rest is exactly that: *your version*. It may be listening to a podcast while lying on your balcony in the sun, reading a novel curled up on your couch, running with your dogs on the beach, enjoying an exercise class like hot yoga with friends, or listening to music while taking a sauna. It might be alone or with someone else. It might be very active or very passive. It might be any combination of these, or something else entirely! And it might change day-to-day. Being flexible and listening to what you need in the moment is key to restoration.

I personally love what actor Sam Waterston says about slowing down and resting to restore: "More and more, the things that give me joy have to do with stopping."[3] For Waterston, his job became a source of pain that affected his mental space and ability to rest and enjoy life, so he quit. "When I did finally quit, I was amazed by the amount of space the job had been taking up in my head. . . . A big piece of myself that I didn't even know I'd rented out is mine again."[4]

Now, I am not saying you should up and quit your job if you feel tired. Rather, look at what is filling up your "mental space" and how it is impacting you. What can you stop to get back more real estate in your mind and brain so that you can be still and experience more joy in life?

As you ask yourself these questions, pay attention to how your current routine makes you feel. Observe this over several days and write down what you experience. Do you do enough of what brings you joy? What is filling up your mental space? What can you "stop" to make more space for rest and restoration in your life?

5. Practice Self-Regulation Before and During Periods of Rest

You will feel more restored if you prepare yourself mentally before your rest activity and self-regulate your thinking during your periods of rest to make sure you get the most from every moment.

To do this, ask yourself questions like:

- What am I thinking of now?
- Am I ruminating on the past, present, or future?
- Can I solve this issue now? (If yes, then solve it and move on, and if no, then set a later time to deal with it.)
- Do I need to refocus on the "now"?
- Is this bringing me mental peace?

Asking yourself these kinds of questions will help you focus on the quality of your rest versus how much rest you are taking, which, in turn, will help you better rest to restore so that you feel less burned out and overwhelmed.

6. Practice the Art of Subtraction

Take things out of your day rather than adding more things to your schedule. We often think adding more practices or gadgets will lead to better outcomes, but it is often when we remove things from our life that we open up more space for rest and restoration. So, ask yourself this: *What can I take out of my day? What can I delegate to someone else to free up my time?* Remember, an open spot on your schedule doesn't need to be filled!

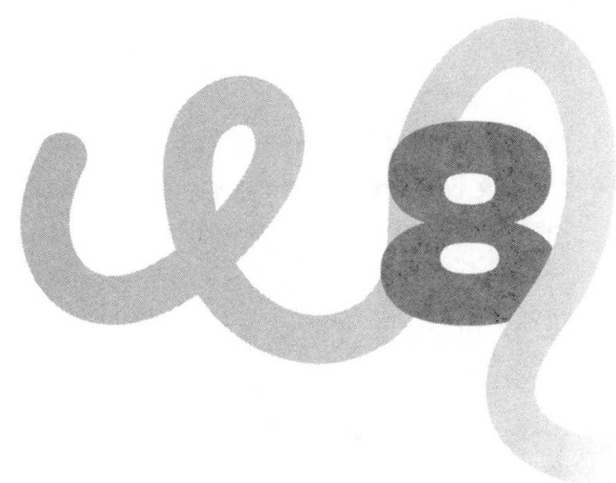

Help, My Intrusive Thoughts Just Won't Quit!

Have you ever watched a hamster run on a wheel? At first, it's fascinating, but after a while, you can't help but feel a little sorry for the hamster. It seems pretty exhausting. When will it stop? Will it go on forever? Should someone help the poor critter out?

It's no wonder we often use this analogy to describe getting stuck in our own heads, especially when it comes to intrusive thoughts. It is so easy to feel like we are trapped, going around and around without end, plagued by images that haunt and overwhelm us.

Intrusive thoughts can be defined as uncontrollable, unwanted thoughts that we feel unable to resist. They feel similar to obsessive-compulsive thinking, where we feel trapped in thinking about the worst thing that could happen or are stuck thinking about something bad that happened to us, replaying this event over and over again, which is similar to negative rumination. And, of course, the more we replay it, the worse and stronger it gets, because whatever we think about the most grows.

This kind of thinking is often a way of handling an underlying unresolved issue. It's not always the most effective or sustainable way to deal with pain or trauma, but it's a kind of coping mechanism—a type of distraction we use to try to keep the source of our pain from crippling us, at least in the short-term. But, as with many coping mechanisms, if left unmanaged it can quickly become a trap itself.

As mentioned in chapter 2, whatever we think about the most is not just random. It's coming from somewhere. Remember, our nonconscious mind absorbs pretty much all (up to about 99 percent) of what we are going through and exposed to. This includes what we read and what's happening in our home, our office, our life, online, politically, culturally, and so on—the good, the bad, and the ugly.

Fortunately, our nonconscious mind scans, evaluates, and neutralizes most of what is in our head. However, because whatever we think about most grows, the more we pay attention to those things, the deeper their roots in our mind grow. They can become intrusive thoughts, and the nonconscious mind will push them into the "waiting room" of the subconscious mind, which, in turn, pushes the most disruptive thought to the front of the queue in our conscious mind as something to be dealt with, as it is hurting our well-being.

Things we have consciously paid attention to on social media, for example; a negative email, text, or call we have thought about a lot; or high–shock value information like the death of a loved one, a dramatic situation in the news, a drama at work, or a sudden emergency can all feed into intrusive thinking habits. Unresolved habits and traumas can also affect our thinking and can influence how intrusive thoughts show up in our life.

If this resonates with you, you are far from alone. The truth is, most of us battle with intrusive thoughts. Research from Concordia University and fifteen other universities worldwide, for example, showed that around 94 percent of people examined across six continents experience unwanted, intrusive thoughts, images, and/or impulses.[1]

Intrusive thoughts are a type of *toxic thought habit*, which is a negative behavioral pattern we have established over time, like getting irritated in traffic, snapping at a loved one, or allowing ourselves to go down worry "rabbit holes" by focusing on a cycle of the negative implications. Whatever we think about the most grows because we give it energy, which, in turn, can negatively impact our overall health and our ability to manage our thoughts both in the moment when we are overwhelmed and in the long-term.

As mentioned, the brain is neuroplastic. This means it is constantly changing. We merge with our environments through our choices, including how long we decide to spend on an intrusive thought. This is why not dealing with intrusive thoughts can literally paralyze our imagination, inhibiting success in school, life, and work, because they are creating negative reinforcing feedback loops. We can hijack our conscious mind, with our messy mind blocking access to our wise nonconscious mind—yes, we can hijack our mind with our mind! This will definitely make us feel like we are constantly trapped on a hamster wheel of intrusive thinking, which itself can become a toxic mindset.

But, as I also mentioned at the beginning of this book, there is always hope. If our brain can change in one direction, it can heal in another. Because our mind is our driving force, and we control our mind, we have a lot of power over how we relate to what has happened to us and how the experiences we have had play out into our future. We can change our mind, brain, and body for the better, even if we have developed an intrusive thought mindset.

And one of the most powerful ways we can do this is by befriending our intrusive thoughts. Yes, you read that correctly! Intrusive thoughts are not just never-ending hamster wheels of pain and anxiety. They can also be windows into our mind, helping us find areas in our life that are problematic so we can change them and heal. They are warning signals that point to things that need addressing so they do not become bigger issues that disrupt our mental and physical well-being.

Think of how a best friend acts. They tell you the truth in a kind and caring way, even if it hurts. And that's how you know they are your best friend: They want the best for you instead of just wanting to please you. They are not doing this to hurt you but to help you heal and be better. This is how you want to start seeing your intrusive thoughts! What are they trying to tell you to help you heal?

Learning how to "be" with yourself and befriend your thoughts is key. This does not mean you will never be sad, unhappy, angry, upset, anxious, or so on. These are normal human emotions we all experience that need to be accepted and managed, not suppressed or ignored. It can be hard to embrace such thoughts and feelings as friends, but it is worth the effort. You can become your own true friend who listens without judgment and is kind and caring, encouraging yourself to keep on keeping on.

This is not going to suddenly take away all your anxieties and pain, but it's the "help in a hurry" first step when you feel overwhelmed by your own thoughts. You can use the information they provide to move forward and, over time, to change and heal.[2]

What I definitely *don't* recommend is suppressing or ignoring your intrusive thoughts. As the adage goes, "What you resist will persist." You cannot heal or overcome what you don't acknowledge or face head-on.

You also cannot simply swap in a more positive thought in place of an intrusive one. The key thing about intrusive thoughts is that they are just that, intrusive. No matter how positive we try to be, they just keep coming back. And the more we try to push the positive, the more we may end up gaslighting our own fears, pain, and trauma, which are often at the root of intrusive thinking, as mentioned above.

In fact, learning how to be alone with our thoughts, even the intrusive ones, is an invaluable mental health skill. When we befriend them, they can provide valuable and potent insight into how we are functioning and what may be impacting our mental and physical well-being and they can positively influence our judgment and decisions.

So, how do you befriend your intrusive thoughts? Below are two simple yet really helpful strategies you can use when you find your thoughts are driving you bananas in the moment.

1. Practice an "I Can" Mindset

One of the greatest gifts you can give to yourself is an "I can help myself deal with my mind" mindset, which will free you to rely on your intuition and strengths that reside in your wise nonconscious mind when no one or nothing else is there to support you. Of course, we all need community, and there is absolutely nothing wrong with asking for help (in fact, it's absolutely necessary in life). However, no matter how many great, loving, wise, and supportive conversations you have with loved ones, friends, therapists, and so on, no one except you can get in your mind (with your mind) to manage the messiness and find out what you need to move forward.

The only person with you 24/7 is yourself—not your therapist, friend, or family member—and you need to know how to handle those alone moments when you feel trapped on that mental hamster wheel. This will take time to learn, but it is possible. Your mind is incredibly powerful and capable, even if it doesn't feel like it at times!

But what does the "I can help myself deal with my mind" mindset look like? It looks like being honest and vulnerable and authentic with yourself. It looks like facing your pain. It looks like being able to sit with the fear, terror, frustration, or whatever other emotions your thoughts dredge up. It looks like seeing the behaviors associated with these emotions and how they have impacted your life. It looks like evaluating how this has messed with or shifted your perspectives and acknowledging how this has affected your mind and health.

Most importantly, it looks like deeply reflecting on *why* this is and finding the source. It looks like deconstructing—and most importantly, reconstructing—the reasons behind why this issue is in your life and how you will find healing. It looks like accepting what has happened and making a decision to reconceptualize and move forward. It looks like deciding how you want your life to play out into your future despite what has happened to you in the past. You are telling yourself you "can" deal with this!

Here are some simple questions that can help you establish this mindset in your life:

1. Acknowledge how your thoughts are impacting you. How do you feel mentally and physically?

2. Why do you think you feel this way? Writing this down can help you organize your thoughts.
3. What do you feel your thoughts are trying to tell you? How can you make them your "friend"? How can you shift your mindset from "I can't deal with this" to "I can face and manage these thoughts"?

For example, say you are a new parent and you are experiencing a lot of intrusive thoughts about all the harm that could come to your child. You worry about them falling down the stairs, hurting themselves badly while trying to walk, or choking on food as they start learning to eat solids. Perhaps these thoughts feel so overwhelming in the moment that you have an anxiety attack, complete with heart palpitations and a sick-to-your-stomach feeling.

First, the key thing would be to acknowledge what these thoughts are and how they are impacting you. Then, question them: What are they trying to tell you? Why do you think you are having these thoughts? Try to see them in a different light. Parents of young children are constantly on alert, as they should be, because there are so many things that can harm children as they are learning to navigate the world, especially when they are so young and vulnerable. Shift this into an "I can" mindset: Instead of letting these thoughts make you feel like you cannot be a good parent, acknowledge them and see them as making you aware of what is happening around you so that you *can* be a better parent.

These intrusive thoughts, although they are stressful, are warning you to be extra careful when you sense a potential threat. They are screaming *Danger! Danger!* and putting you in a state of good stress so that you are ready to protect your child and take action. They are not just thoughts of horrible things that can happen but signals for you to pay attention so these horrible things *do not* happen to your child. Your mind is merely reminding you that you can and should protect your baby from things that can seriously hurt them, and you do this by paying closer attention to your surroundings. It's got your back so you can be the best parent you can be in the moment.

2. Counter Intrusive Thoughts with Deliberate Thinker Moments

As mentioned in chapter 7, thinker moments, where we just take some time to daydream and let our mind wander, aren't just an odd mental quirk. They are a natural and spontaneous way to teach ourselves how to live a self-examined life. And, as our mind wanders and thoughts become intrusive, practicing thinker moments can help us examine what we are thinking about and our own experiences.

Contrary to popular belief, the mind does not grind to a halt when we are daydreaming. It activates the coexisting default mode network (DMN) and task positive network (TPN) in the brain in a constructive and healthy way.[3] The DMN is a primary network that we switch into when we switch off from the outside world and move into a state of focused mindfulness, which is a great way to train our mind to avoid falling into a state of toxic stress when we experience intrusive thinking.

The TPN, on the other hand, supports the active thinking required for making healthy decisions. So, as we focus our thinking and activate the DMN, at some point in our thinking process we move into active decision-making. This activates the TPN, which helps us face our intrusive thoughts, see what they are trying to tell us, and make them our friend.

Here's how to use a thinker moment when you find yourself getting stuck on the hamster wheel of intrusive thinking:

1. Switch off to the external and switch on to the internal by closing your eyes and focusing on the detail of what is going through your mind. Observe this for around sixty seconds.
2. Next, open your eyes and tell yourself out loud what you have just thought about.
3. Try to distinguish between the thoughts that are free-flowing and the thoughts that are getting stuck, which you keep finding yourself coming back to.
4. For the latter, evaluate whether these thoughts were giving you a sense of peace or making you upset or concerned.
5. Step into "friend mode," where you see yourself as a kind, compassionate, understanding, and nonjudgmental friend to your thoughts.
6. Give yourself an alternate way of thinking about these thoughts to help reframe your perspective in the moment, like the example used above. Don't try to solve this problem. Just focus on what you need to say to yourself in *this* moment to help you get to the *next* moment. This doesn't have to be a positive version of the thought; it's more of another way of seeing it, or another perspective. It could be something as simple as "I did my best in that situation," "It is hard to grieve, and that's okay," "Maybe I could have done something differently, but I can't change the past," or "What's behind me doesn't matter as much as what I can do going forward." (You can use the table below for this step.)

7. If you can't think of anything in the moment, you could simply say "I recognize I am stuck, and I am going to ask a friend/someone I trust what they think about how I should manage this situation." Don't be afraid to reach out and ask for help! We all need help at times, especially when it comes to our thinking.
8. Don't let yourself marinate in your thinking. Try to move on by repeating this phrase, or your reframed thought, as many times as you need to so that you do not go back to that negative space of mind.

Use the following table to practice this, create your own table, or use the QR code at the end of the chapter to download it.

My Thinker Moment	
What did I just think?	
Was that thought free-flowing or stuck?	
What direction is my mind going in?	

Am I in a kind, compassionate, and nonjudgmental space toward myself?	
If not, how can I get there? **Where do I think this thought is coming from?**	
What's an alternative way of looking at this thought?	

Here is an example of what this could look like:

What did I just think? *I am going to mess up and embarrass myself at work. I keep seeing this happen in my mind and can't stop thinking about how horrible things are going to go.*

Was that thought free-flowing or stuck? *Stuck.*

What direction is my mind going in? *I keep seeing myself do something embarrassing. I am even dreaming about this every night!*

Am I in a kind, compassionate, and nonjudgmental space toward myself? If not, how can I get there? *No. Maybe I can talk to someone I trust to get perspective. I can also try to think of all the things I have gotten right in my life. I am not always a mess-up! And it is okay to fail—we all fail at times.*

Where do I think this thought is coming from? *In the past, I messed up and still cringe from how embarrassed I felt at that moment. Even now, thinking about it, I feel sick to my stomach and just want to hide forever.*

What's an alternative way of looking at this thought? *I need to remind myself that we all do embarrassing things sometimes. This makes us human! I will think of times other people have embarrassed themselves in front of me. I did not think it was the end of the world, and I did not judge that person harshly. I just thought it was a very human thing to do. I know I am more nervous about this upcoming workweek because I have an important project I don't want to mess up. I have prepared as much as I can and worked hard on this project. The only thing I can do is give it my best! I can't control for all circumstances, but this doesn't mean I will just embarrass myself and everyone will laugh at me.*

When doing this exercise, remember that friends tend to give us helpful information about ourselves. So, when you experience an intrusive thought, pause and try to really step into your "friend zone." Imagine a friend has come to you with this problem. What would you say to them?

This often helps us be more honest with ourselves, which, when we have identified what is really bothering us, allows us to be more compassionate with ourselves and what we are going through instead of adding to our stress. It is like pulling back the curtain and finding the Wizard of Oz is just a regular person!

To download the table from this chapter, visit helpinahurrybook.com/resources

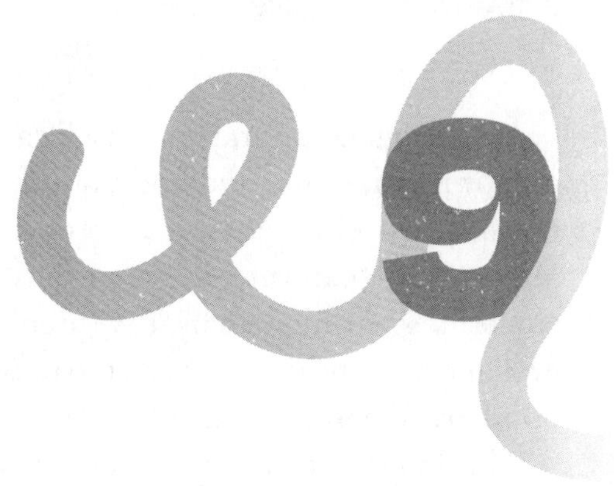

Help, I Don't Feel Happy All the Time!

When we're scrolling through social media, it is easy to believe that happiness is what we are all searching for—a "happiness" that usually consists of us smiling in front of commodities like money or fancy cars, or even from getting likes on a picture. Marketing ads for new products almost always mention "happiness" as an end goal, whether we are watching an advertisement for a new soda, new holiday, or new drug. Smiling, happy people stare at us from billboards as we drive to work or walk around our neighborhood—there is no escaping them. Life is all about happiness . . . right?

Often, it feels like happiness and positivity are touted as the wonder drug to solve our problems. It is easy to feel like there is something wrong with us if we are not as happy as other people seem to be! Yet these images, online and in real life, only show the highlights. No one wants to post their down or messy moments for all the world to see.

Yes, being happy and optimistic can have a positive impact on our mind, brain, and body, but thinking happy thoughts doesn't just eliminate whatever we are going through—although we can certainly be excused if we think there is something wrong with us if we aren't happy all the time, or even most of the time. That's the message so many of us are bombarded with every day, so it must mean something, right?

Thinking in healthy ways does most certainly have a positive impact on our mind, brain, and body, but it's not a simple thought swap or mindset shift. Nor is it something we need to do all the time. Just thinking happy thoughts doesn't eliminate whatever we are going through or make life easier.

To truly heal and find some measure of lasting, intrinsic happiness, we must move beyond positive affirmations and thinking and face what is holding us back through embracing, processing, and reconceptualizing our past pain. If we don't do this, we won't truly benefit from positive psychology and happiness techniques. Using the latter before we have processed and managed what has happened to us often results in a toxic positivity cycle, where we feel bad for simply being human, try to ignore our more uncomfortable emotions, and discover it only makes us feel worse.

In fact, research indicates that pursuing happiness in a toxically positive way can impact our ability to fully embrace the human experience, with all its ups and downs and uncertainties. Our life is infused with fragility, setbacks, and unpredictability as much as it is filled with passion, excitement, and joy. Using happiness or positive thinking to mask the harsh realities of life will backfire because there is no avoiding what it means to be human.

It is okay *not* to feel okay.[1] It is okay not to be happy all the time. An adverse emotional response to an adverse life situation is normal. Understandably, we don't want to get stuck in a dark, negative place, but happiness is not a bandage we can slap on all of life's wounds and just "keep on keeping on." Happiness is an important part of living, yes, but it will not take away the pain we experience as we go through life.

Not only is it okay to *not* feel okay, but it is an essential part of what it means to be human. An adverse emotional response to an adverse situation is normal and healthy.[2] Think of soldiers coming back from war. If they did not feel some level of unhappiness at what they saw and experienced, we would question their humanity.

Happiness also means different things to different people. How we understand happiness, or the social and cultural ideations of happiness we are exposed to, are just "one slice of humanity's cultural diversity."[3] Broadly speaking, *failing* to feel happy all the time is more of a concern in Western philosophy, while *feeling* happy all the time is more of a concern in Eastern philosophy. Western cultures often seem to associate happiness with having positive feelings all or at least most of the time and with accumulating "things."

Eastern cultures, on the other hand, tend to associate the pursuit of happiness with worse well-being and poor character development and believe the pursuit of peace and embracing the downs of life as necessary lessons are healthier for a person's well-being. And logically, the socioeconomic and political factors, weather, and disease prevalence and management where we live of course play into our sense of happiness too.

Moreover, it appears that feelings of happiness aren't as common as we are led to believe. Most of the time, we actually *don't* feel okay.[4] Generally, we are literally just going through the day, dealing with the ups and downs of life in a fairly neutral state, with occasional bursts of happiness, irritation, frustration, and so on. Michael Linden, an expert in mood disorders and a professor of psychiatry at the Charité University Hospital in Berlin, notes that

> even a moment's reflection about daily life reveals that a feeling of happiness is actually pretty rare. We spend much of our time simply "OK," trying to ignore that we're feeling a little tired, run down, upset, stressed out, irritated or in pain, straining to stay on task and manage our responsibilities.[5]

A strong desire to be happy all the time can actually reduce our sense of well-being.[6] The idealization of happiness can throw us into a state of negative rumination, where we can quickly get stuck going round in endless circles questioning why we are not happy when we are doing everything that is supposed to make us happy. This, in turn, can lead to disappointment in oneself for having a "low mood," which, research shows, comes from the *over*valuation of happiness. This, in turn, creates a discrepancy between so-called ideal happiness and "actual or realistic happiness."[7] Bottom line: In pursuing happiness, we run the risk of being even more depressed and then feeling guilty about it—and a vicious cycle is quickly set up.

Interestingly, happiness and well-being tend to go hand in hand when we are more focused on socially engaged paths to happiness than individual gains or possessions.[8] This pairs well with the findings of one of the world's longest happiness studies, which showed that "relationships in all their forms—friendships, romantic partnerships, families, coworkers, tennis partners, book club members, Bible study groups—all contribute to a happier, healthier life."[9]

Even if all our happiness dreams came true, this does not mean we would actually be happy all the time. Often, when we feel happy, we still wish we could be even *happier*, which can lead to increased feelings of anxiety and sadness. Research shows that if happiness is perceived as an important or even major life goal—where "happiness" is equated to constant feelings of happiness that result in a preoccupation about feeling happy—this can potentially increase our chances of experiencing depression.[10] If we value happiness too much, we may end up harming our mental health. True, lasting happiness is perhaps best described as the ability to tolerate unhappiness.

Indeed, chasing after happiness can make time feel scarce. Several studies have indicated that trying to be happy all the time tends to make people feel like time is running out, which, paradoxically, makes them stressed out and unhappy![11] If happiness is our only goal in life, and if we constantly feel the need to be happy, we can quickly lose our ability to appreciate and treasure each moment of our life for what it is: time we will never get back.

One of the biggest mistakes many of us make is viewing happiness as a destination, a noun. With this thinking, we get stuck in the idea that "If I just do *x* I will be happy," instead of seeing that lasting happiness is a state of motion, a verb. It is the sum of our moments rather than any particular place, person, or state.

If you feel pressured to be happy all the time, take the time to pause and examine your thoughts. Ask yourself:

- Is the happiness fallacy taking up mental real estate in my mind?
- Do I feel guilty when I feel unhappy?
- Do I think there is something wrong with me when I feel sad, upset, or angry?

- Do I feel shame, guilt, and embarrassment if I don't feel happy all the time?
- Do I often tell myself (and others) that I just need to "think a positive/happy thought" if I am feeling sad, angry, or any emotion that is considered uncomfortable or negative?
- Do I find myself ignoring or repressing my suffering or pain?

If you answered yes to any or all of these, you can work on reframing how you see happiness and its role in your life. Here are some action tips to help you practice this in your life.

1. Listen to Your Thoughts as If You Were Talking to a Friend

Don't let your guilt consume you; rather, be curious, almost as if you were listening to a friend tell you about their thoughts. When you find yourself falling into a pattern of using toxic positivity to suppress your more uncomfortable emotions, pause and ask yourself, *Why do I feel the way I do?* Examine the "why" behind your thinking. How do you understand happiness? What has shaped your views on happiness?

Next, say out loud: "Not only is it okay for me not to feel okay, it is part of what it means to be human, and trying to be happy all the time can hurt me and make my pain worse." Remind yourself of this at least seven times a day, for as many days as possible, to make this your new mindset. You can set this as a notification on your device or write it on sticky notes placed around your workstation/desk/home. Whatever works for you!

2. Shift from State Orientation to Action Orientation

Embracing an "action orientation" mindset is immensely helpful if you feel the 100 percent happiness fallacy creeping in and impacting your mental health. An action orientation mindset means being able to focus on a task without being preoccupied or even sabotaged by the thoughts swirling through your mind with their attached emotions, behaviors, bodily sensations, and perspectives. The thoughts don't disappear, but you focus on what needs to be done in that moment rather than what is swirling around in your head. This is kind of like compartmentalization and is a helpful skill that can be beneficial in many areas of your life.

This mindset is the opposite of immersing yourself in a "state orientation" mindset, which focuses on thinking about how you feel in the moment; for example, paying attention to thoughts like: *Why am I not 100 percent happy right now? What's wrong with me? Why can't I just swap the bad for the good?* An action orientation mindset will help you accomplish the task at hand, whereas a state orientation mindset can quickly lead to rumination and feelings of sadness and dissatisfaction.

To practice this, give yourself around five seconds to acknowledge (but not dwell on) what you are thinking about, with its accompanying feelings. Remind yourself that this is just how you're feeling right now—it is your state orientation mindset. Next, observe how this is making you feel. For example, distracted, preoccupied, and maybe even a little anxious or edgy. You can write this down to help you organize your thoughts and feelings in the moment.

Now, shift to an action orientation mindset by choosing to focus on a specific task that redirects your attention. For example, you can choose to finish that work task, clean that area of the house you have been putting off, bake that new recipe, go out for coffee with that friend or colleague, do that online yoga class, or whatever works to help you shift your focus.

It may take some time to get into this task or action, and that is okay. You are working on shifting your attention and focus, which can take time when your thoughts are particularly demanding. Don't worry or give up if you don't do this well at first!

3. Use Go-To Sayings to Keep a "Happy" Balance

It can be helpful to have a go-to phrase or saying you practice thinking about every day to change how you perceive happiness and its role in your life.

I love these two phrases, which are used in Finland and Denmark, places that consistently rank the highest in happiest countries globally.[12] They reflect mindsets of facing, embracing, processing, and reconceptualizing what life throws our way and are not simple affirmations or positive statements:

Whatever you leave behind you, you will find in front of you. This saying suggests that suppressing or avoiding things from your past can make them worse, and they will come back to haunt you in the future. You can try to pursue happiness in the moment, but you should not do this at the expense of your future by avoiding your more uncomfortable or "unhappy" emotions. What you ignore doesn't just disappear. To be truly happy, you have to embrace unhappiness as well.

Some have happiness; everyone has summer. This saying suggests that no matter what you are facing and going through right now, it will pass. Just as happy moments do not last, sad moments also have an expiration date—summer will come soon. Better days are ahead!

To these two statements I would also add:

Being unhappy doesn't mean I have an unhappy life. When stuck in what feels like an "unhappy pit," remind yourself that this moment will pass. You have gotten through many low moments in life before.

You can start with just these three statements, or you can create a bigger list of phrases or sayings that resonate with you, which you can keep to remind yourself that happiness is more than the feeling of being happy in the moment. Put them where you will see them: on your fridge, in your car, as a reminder on your phone, or whatever works for you.

4. Embrace Community

We are social beings: Our mind and brain thrive when we are part of a community, while isolation can wreak havoc on our mental and physical health.[13] When we are isolated, our cortisol levels rise, which can cause low-grade inflammation across the brain and body, making us feel ill, reducing blood flow to the brain, and upsetting our mental clarity and our mood—isolation literally makes us lose our perspective.

When we connect with others, however, our brain and body respond in a positive way, healing our body and reducing cortisol levels and inflammation while protecting the heart and immune system.[14] Indeed, community can be "addictive." The mesolimbic dopamine system, a system linked to addiction, lights up when we reach out and give to others, providing us with a deep sense of happiness.

This is why it is so important to make an effort to reach out and connect with the people around you, even if you identify as an introvert. We all need some level of support and community. You need to tune in, not just say hello and carry on with your life.

Not only should you be okay with asking for help or companionship but you also need to be aware of what the people around you are going through and reach out to help them, switching off to yourself, even if this just means listening to someone and being there for them as they cry.

This is incredibly powerful and can have a remarkable effect on our mental well-being and overall sense of happiness and fulfillment. The more we reach out to others, the more we actually help ourselves. Deep, meaningful relationships help us communicate and deal with our feelings rather than suppressing them. In these kinds of relationships, we feel safe; we can be open about what we are going through. This helps us face our issues rather than ignoring them, which will only make us ill and affect our mental health. And when we communicate openly with others about what we are going through, neurotransmitters like serotonin and dopamine start flowing, which help heal the brain and body, give us insight, develop our perspective, and make us happy. Even just a hug releases hormones that make us feel calmer, valued, and happier.

And there are so many ways to become part of a community:

- Volunteer at a local nonprofit.
- Attend or start a book club, or any kind of club that sounds interesting.
- Start your own meetup group.

- Have lunch with your colleagues.
- Join a sports league.
- Schedule a lunch, dinner, or coffee date with a friend or family member on a weekly basis.
- Schedule monthly video chats if you live far away from a friend or loved one.
- Check out sites like Meetup or Timeleft, or find groups in your area that organize weekly or monthly dinners with strangers.

The possibilities are endless.

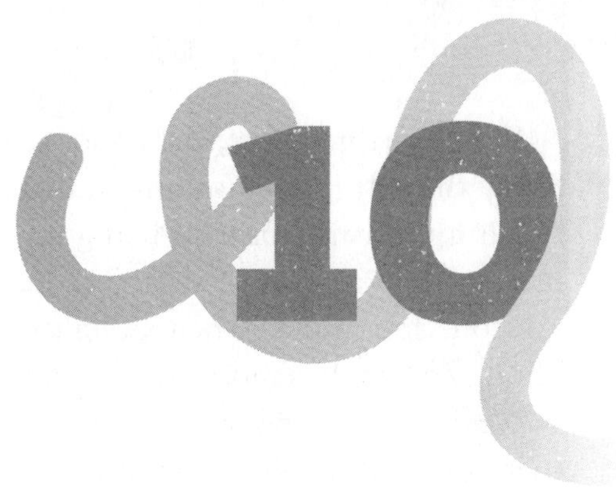

Help, I'm Angry All the Time!

Anger is a complex emotion. It can be helpful but also harmful. It can be chaotic or can serve a purpose—when we learn how to manage and harness it. The key here is frequency. An occasional outburst won't cripple you, and may even be necessary at times, depending on the circumstances. It's the frequency over time that we have to watch out for.

An important part of managing anger is understanding what an emotion is. Every moment of every day, we are thinking, feeling, and choosing. This happens in response to what we experience while awake. This activity builds actual physical thoughts inside the brain and impacts the body down to the cellular level, as well as the mind energy, as mentioned in chapter 2.

Remember, your thoughts look like trees. The branches of these trees contain the product of your thinking, feeling, and choosing (your mind-in-action). Emotions are like the leaves of these trees; they have a physical and chemical structure in the brain. They are produced by your mind.

When we think, feel, and choose, we experience emotion. Every thought has emotional information attached to it—this is an intrinsic part of being human. So, every thought has emotion as part of its structure, which is stored in the nonconscious mind. When thoughts move into the conscious mind, we feel the emotions of them.

We cannot escape our emotions, and we cannot suppress them. If we do, they can explode in other areas of our life. This is true for anger. It is a normal emotion we all feel and is not bad in and of itself. It can motivate us—but it can also hinder us if left unmanaged, like a volcano waiting to erupt.

Typical things that can make us angry are traffic jams, arrogant or rude people, being yelled at, someone who wastes our time, having to wait too long for something, feeling like we have been "used," being lied to, being unjustly punished or wrongfully accused, having too much on our plate, or not dealing with our emotions.

I think we can all recall a time when we were justifiably angry and a time when we let our anger get the better of us—usually when we were stressed, overwhelmed, or burned out. Recently, I was getting into bed when I glanced at my emails and saw a bunch of things I had missed during the course of the day—tasks I really needed to do, even though I just wanted to sleep. This made me really angry, which led to an outburst that my husband was, unfortunately, on the other end of. At that moment, things felt so overwhelming and I was so angry I just wanted to run away and hide from everything and everyone.

I got so frustrated and negative that I shocked myself. I realized these types of angry outbursts were becoming a pattern in my life. Yes, I had a lot on my plate, and this may have excused some of my behavior, but it was not healthy in the short- or long-term. So, in that moment, I stopped, stepped back metaphorically, and observed myself and my behavior. I rewound back to when my angry outbursts more or less began, looked for their potential origin, triggers, and frequency, and recognized I needed help in a hurry before this became a bigger problem in my life.

Research has shown that repeated angry outbursts can add up, not only making us pretty miserable to be around but also creating disorder in the mind, brain, and body if left unmanaged.[1] Anger primes our body's fight-or-flight response, which results in the following:

- The adrenal glands release a flood of stress hormones like adrenaline and cortisol into the body.
- The brain shunts blood away from the gut and toward our muscles in preparation for physical exertion.
- Our heart rate and blood pressure increase while our breathing gets more rapid in preparation for a fight-or-flight response.
- We experience a rise in body temperature and increased perspiration.

This response is okay, in short bursts, if caused by "healthy" anger. It sharpens the mind and brain so that we can achieve a goal, such as defending ourselves from an unjust attack. Revving us up, so to speak, this response can help channel our energy in a productive way.

However, if it's unhealthy anger, such as road rage, or anger that is left unmanaged over time, this fight-or-flight response becomes distorted, and the constant flood of stress chemicals and associated metabolic changes can cause harm to many different systems in the brain and body, affecting our mental and physical health.

Again, it's the frequency over time that we have to watch out for. Just one or two angry outbursts a day over several weeks (around 63 days[2]) can create an established habit, or negative coping mechanism, in our life.

Because emotion and cognition are so dynamically linked to bodily arousal—the mind-brain-body connection—when we are angry, even nonconsciously, this will affect the *way* our mind, brain, and body prioritize resources, favoring action states at the expense of clear thinking, decision-making, and choice of words.[3] When we frequently become angry in this way, it not only impairs our ability to think well and make good decisions but also our health, as the body produces numerous proteins and hormones that increase inflammation, which can raise our risk of many diseases.

In fact, a lot of bad things can start happening in the brain if we are chronically angry. We tend to get more and more headaches, and, over time, increase our risk of a stroke. The attention and visual processing areas of the brain also get more active than normal, affecting our overall brain health.[4] Angry outbursts put the amygdala, which is like a library holding our emotional perceptions and information on associations between experiences and emotions, into an overactive state. When this happens, it's a bit like running through a library and illogically grabbing books chaotically all over the place, impacting our ability to think, process emotions and experiences, and function over time.[5]

Frequent angry outbursts can affect the blood vessels of the heart, potentially increasing our risk for heart disease.[6] This happens because uncontrolled anger causes an increase of stress hormones called catecholamines, which increase blood pressure and play a role in the development of artery-clogging plaque, which, over the course of years, can lead to coronary artery disease. However, even a sudden surge of catecholamines during fits of anger can cause heart attacks, lethal heart rhythms, or rapid weakening of the heart muscle itself, a condition known as stress cardiomyopathy or broken heart syndrome.[7]

Our gastrointestinal (GI) tract is also very sensitive to our emotions since it is connected to our brain's hypothalamus. It also controls feelings of satiety and hunger, which means that unmanaged anger can upset our ability to eat and digest food as well as upset our emotional state of mind, impacting the release of the neuropeptides in the gut and the assimilation of nutrients.

Additionally, as mentioned above, anger activates the body's sympathetic nervous system, or fight-or-flight system, which moves blood away from the gut to major muscles.[8] This slows down movement in the GI tract, which can lead to problems like gaps between cells in the lining of the intestines, which means food and waste can get in and create inflammation that can cause symptoms such as stomach pain, bloating, or constipation. We are seeing more and more research on this link between emotional mind states and GI issues.

So, to say that it is worth "catching" those angry outbursts before they make things worse is a bit of an understatement. We set ourselves up for all kinds of issues when we let our anger control us rather than learning how to manage our anger in the moment.

Of course, this is so much easier said than done, as angry outbursts are just that: sudden, intense bursts of emotion that often leave us blindsided in the moment. So, to help you process and manage these, here are several strategies you can use in the moment so your anger doesn't become a habit that negatively impacts your well-being.

1. Observe If It's a Pattern or One-Off

The first thing to do is to observe if this is a pattern in your life or something that only happens occasionally. Here are some questions you can ask yourself to determine this over several days or a week:

- How often are you having angry outbursts? Daily? Multiple times a day? Almost daily?
- Is there a particular time of day this happens?
- Is there a particular person, place, or situation triggering these angry outbursts?
- Have people commented that you seem more angry and irritable than normal?
- Has there been some unexpected change in your life recently that has upset you and has potentially made you feel out of control?

You can write these questions down to help keep track of what you are observing. It is also useful to know the early signs of uncontrolled anger, which include a faster heart rate, muscle tension, clenched fists, or racing thoughts. By identifying these signs early, you can learn how to intervene and manage your emotions before your anger escalates.

2. Give Yourself Space

If you're feeling intensely angry, step away from the situation that triggered the anger. Take a break to cool off and gain perspective before addressing the issue. It is okay to let someone know that you just need some time to decompress before you respond. Put your mental and physical health first!

A great way to do this is to practice deep breathing for a few moments. I love using the ten-second pause exercise:

- Take a really deep breath in for two counts, feeling your rib cage expand outward.
- Hold for two counts.
- Now, force the air out with a whooshing sound for six counts.
- Repeat this, but now add the word *let* and stretch it out when you breathe in for two counts and hold for two counts, then add the word *go* and stretch it out slowly over your six-count exhale. You can do this out loud or silently in your mind. You are essentially saying "let go" over a ten-second period. You can repeat this sequence as many times and as often as you need to!

The ten-second pause is a great way to start regulating angry outbursts because it helps you calm down your neurophysiological responses to anger in the moment, which is important because the highly sensory nature of anger can create a feedback loop that is hard to exit once it begins. The way our body feels when we are angry almost serves to spur the anger on.

You can also use this excellent breathing exercise to lower your blood pressure in the moment:

- Breathe in for six counts.
- Breathe out for six counts.
- Do this six times.
- I recommend repeating this sequence up to four times.

3. Change How You Respond

When you're ready to address the issue, you want to communicate your feelings calmly and assertively, not make assumptions about the other person's intentions. Use "I" statements to express how you feel without blaming or accusing others. For example, say, "I felt hurt when . . ." rather than "You made me angry when . . ."

The best way to do this is to think about what you are going to say and practice using this kind of language when you are *not* angry so it becomes an ingrained habit over time. It can be useful in so many situations and relationships, especially when you need to defuse an argument or tense conversation.

4. Shift Your Mindset

Once you have calmed down, think about how you can reframe your angry outburst. Shift your mind from *This is why I'm angry* to *How can I see it differently in this moment?* and *What can I do about this?* Instead of dwelling on your anger, focus on finding solutions. Ask yourself what you can do to address the situation or prevent similar issues in the future. And remember to ask for help with this if you feel you need it. This proactive approach can help redirect your energy in a productive way.

You can do this by replacing negative and hostile thoughts with more rational and balanced ones. For example, replace *I hate these people* with *I hate what these people are doing and how it affects me. Perhaps I can communicate this in some way.*

It is also helpful to ask yourself in the moment if your anger is proportional to the situation. Is it justified? If yes, then why? What can you do about it? If not, then how can you work on your responses? Get comfortable with questioning yourself and your own intentions—this is a really helpful skill in so many situations.

5. Look for the Underlying Cause

Often, frequent anger is a sign of either deep sadness or deep fear. To find what may be at the root of your anger, observe who makes you angry or what scenarios make you angry. What is the common theme? Perhaps it's the fear of what may happen if you fail, so you get angry if people don't perform up to your standard. Perhaps it's the sadness you feel when you lose a sense of freedom or sense of stability—this grief can manifest as anger. By working through my Neurocycle app, you just may find a surprising reason behind your anger.

To download the Neurocycle app, visit www.neurocycle.app

5. Look for the Underlying Cause

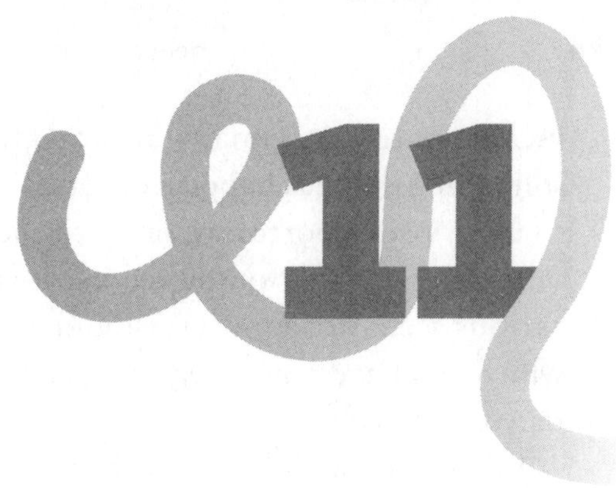

Help, My Regrets Are Holding Me Back!

Whenever I think of regrets, the opening words of Florence and the Machine's song "Shake It Out" come to mind, where she sings about regrets collecting like old friends. Unmanaged regret can make us feel like we are truly wading through a swamp with no end in sight. It is one of those emotions that is so crippling that it can be hard to get through the day, let alone move forward or heal. It is so easy to feel like we are drowning in our "darkest moments."

Regret is also pretty insidious. It tends to haunt so many areas of our life at once, sometimes without us even realizing until it is too late. Suddenly, we are caught in a thunderstorm of disappointment, guilt, remorse, sorrow, or helplessness and are left asking how, exactly, we got here and how we can leave.

Regret encompasses so many human emotions, mainly sadness, disappointment, and frustration, and can leave us incapacitated and unable to heal. It usually results from something that has happened, something that has been done to us, a lost opportunity, or lost time. We tend to take out our regrets mostly on ourselves, torturing our mind with various scenarios on what should or could have happened, which can have many negative mental and physical health repercussions.

Regret feels awful because, by its nature, it makes us think there *was* something we could have done or said differently or some better choice we could have made. It compounds all these swirling emotions with feelings of guilt and shame, further incapacitating our ability to move on and heal.[1]

Over time, this can impact our overall well-being because the emotional distress that unmanaged regret triggers can dysregulate our hormones and immune system, making them vulnerable to ill-health.[2] Imaging studies show increased activity in areas of the brain called the medial orbitofrontal cortex, the anterior cingulate cortex, and the hippocampus when we experience regret.[3] If we stay in this state of mind, this high activity can become unbalanced and contribute to all kinds of problems in the brain and body.

Regret is a type of counterfactual thinking, or "could have/would have/should have" thinking.[4] It focuses on what might have been or alternatives to something that has happened in the past and is something we all experience at some time or another.[5] Regrets are reconstructions of "what might have been" with a mixture of facts and imagined scenarios based on the proverbial "if."

There are two main types of could have/would have/should have thinking. The first, *upward counterfactuals*, are better alternatives: imagining a more positive outcome if we had done something differently in the past, making what occurred seem more negative. For example, "If I had taken that job, I would have been happier." *Downward counterfactuals*, on the other hand, are imaginings of worse alternatives, making what actually occurred seem more positive.[6] For instance, "If I had taken that road, I could have been injured in that accident."

Research shows that downward counterfactuals can have better psychological effects than upward counterfactuals, but the key is *balance*.[7] Even a downward counterfactual can make us feel worse because we see what could have been, which may make us anxious and upset and can result in a negative rumination spiral on the possible harm that could have happened. However, a balance of upward and downward counterfactual thinking can make us feel more prepared for the future—if we turn what happened into a learning experience. So, regrets are not always negative. They can stir us to positive action; for instance, we may regret not learning a certain skill that we ended up needing, which can then motivate us to do so now and help ourselves in the future.

Regrets are 100 percent normal. Life is packed with choices, many of which go wrong. Even the most "well-lived" life is not perfect. In many ways, regret is inevitable. Some of the most common regrets we experience are ones relating to education, career, romance, parenting, the self, and leisure, which, as we know, are all ongoing and organic experiences filled with choices and possible mistakes.[8] These regrets, if managed, can help us learn from our mistakes by allowing us to see possibilities and potential outcomes, which gives us better data for more informed decisions.[9] Dwelling on the past in a healthy way, to learn something about our current and future selves, can help us conceptualize and realize our "ideal self" in the future as well as help with regret in the present by emphasizing our ability to grow and heal.[10]

It is important to remember that life is a narrative-building process, an unfolding story of experiences, choices, *and* potential regrets. Looking back can help us see that we did the best (or worst) in any given situation, based on the information we had and who we were at the time. It's always a good idea to remember that we made decisions based on the information we had *at the time*, and sometimes the best lesson we can learn from regret is to be realistic about the expectations and limitations we faced in that particular moment and phase of our life.

Contextualizing past decisions in this way can help us gain insight into our regret today, give us a sense of autonomy, and improve our well-being by showing us how we can learn and grow from these experiences as well as how far we have already come in life. This is what I call stepping into "positive regret": using our tendency to dwell on the past to help us prepare for the future. As I always like to say, there are no bad emotions, just information.

Below are several tips to guide you in how to manage your regrets in the moment when you find yourself fixating on your regret to the point it's distracting you from your day-to-day life, keeping you trapped in the past, and impacting your ability to function and your health. These will help you turn these spirals into "positive regret," changing how the past impacts your present and future.

1. Develop a Possibilities Mindset

A possibilities mindset perceives all kinds of possibilities and potentialities in any given situation. It is intrinsically hopeful and can help you reframe regret as a part of your journey toward a future, better destination.

When you embrace a possibilities mindset, you see "could have" and "would have" scenarios as possibilities that may or may not have happened and that provide enriching information that may be useful for yourself or someone else in the future. These regrets become data to augment your experience as opposed to a battering ram to beat yourself up.

Being able to see possibilities in the midst of your regrets is a game-changer. It transforms your thinking, allowing you to keep writing your story. To practice this, don't allow yourself to see your regrets as failures that define who you are as a person. See them as possibilities that didn't materialize, which you can still learn from to open up future probabilities. Visualize these scenarios as opportunities where you gained knowledge that will help you in the future.

To make this a habit, deliberately and intentionally *practice* seeing possibilities in every regret you have and write them down, which will help organize your thinking. Using a table format is a great way to do this. Try to see at least three possibilities for every regret you experience. This will help you start seeing that life is more than just one direction or road.

The more you do this, the more you will find yourself applying these in your life. Start with more simple regrets first to build up your resilience to face any major regrets you have been holding on to.

For example, maybe you are struggling financially as an entrepreneur and find yourself regretting all the things you did wrong or may have done wrong and wondering if your business will survive the next several months. To shift into a "possibilities mindset," you first acknowledge how you feel and why. You notice how you are starting to spiral into regret and how this is making you anxious, upset, and even more overwhelmed.

Next, you write down the regrets you have on one side of a piece of paper or in a document on your computer or device—whatever works for you. For example, "When I contracted a particular company to do a task, I didn't do my due diligence, trusted them too much, and lost money because they ended up overcharging me."

Then, in the center of the page, beside each regret, start writing all the things you have learned from this experience, even if it is only what not to do. For example, you may note down that in the future you need to ask more questions and get procedures, costs, and timelines in writing in advance.

In a third column on the other side of the page, write all the possibilities this regret generates. For example, "I have learned so much, including the need to bring more of the work in-house, which I have done, to save money and increase efficiency in the long-term."

Finally, decide what would help your current situation and what you need to make this start happening. For example, where can you streamline operations to save money and increase profit? What else can you do as you recover your losses?

2. Employ Controlled Indulging

The key to using regret to your advantage is to analyze it but not dwell on it, which is what I mean by *controlled indulging*. While you shouldn't ruminate on regret, you shouldn't ignore it either. Give yourself the space needed to face your regrets, but do not allow yourself to spiral. Set aside a specific time to evaluate a particular regret, then move on with your day. During this time:

- Name the regret out loud (you can also write it down).
- Reflect by asking who, what, how, and why questions. Where is this coming from? Why? How is it affecting you now?

- Try to look at the regret from a different angle, as though you are advising someone else who has this issue. How do you want this to play out in your life? How will you heal and move forward?

The key here is not to keep chewing on your regret. Rather, you need to find a different way to think about it that will help you move forward. Remember that you cannot change what has happened to you, but you can change what happens *in* you. You are in control of the *now*, which means you can control how your past plays into your future.

Some great ways to do this are as follows:

- Find a quote, song, passage, or phrase that inspires you. Put this somewhere you will see it, and read it often, especially when you feel your regrets start to take hold.
- Remind yourself that it's okay to fail, make a mess, and have regrets; you are human, and it is part of the journey of discovery. You are figuring out who you are and what you want, and you are learning so much.
- As much as it hurts and is frustrating, and as much as you might want to turn back the hands of time, try to see every regret you have as an insight into who you are and how you can repair and grow as a person.
- When wading through the pain and frustration of failure and regretting past decisions, we often don't realize what lies ahead, so work on focusing on your future as well. Give yourself permission to hope and dream.
- Tell yourself that the best way to master regret is to embrace it for the message it brings to you as a person.

- Counter regret in the moment with this simple saying: "Don't get stuck trying to make the right decision; make the decision right." This will help remind you that hindsight is 20/20, and all you can do now is make what happened "right" and learn for next time.
- Talk to someone you trust about your regrets. Thoughts and emotions lose their intensity and power when spoken out loud, especially when spoken to someone else, as they can give you a different perspective.

Below is a table to help you organize this information as you learn how to manage the regret you are feeling. You also can create your own, if you want, or use the QR code at the end of the chapter to download it.

Reconceptualizing My Regrets

Regret	What has happened in the past that led to this regret?	What is happening in the present that is leading to this level of regret?	How do I want this regret to influence my future?

Regret	What has happened in the past that led to this regret?	What is happening in the present that is leading to this level of regret?	How do I want this regret to influence my future?

3. Use the Multiple Perspective Advantage

Our decisions tend to be influenced or driven by the strongest emotional memory associated with the strongest thought that has been triggered in that moment. This is how regrets can have so much power over our current decisions, keeping us trapped in the past.

One way to help you deal with this strong emotional push is to practice standing outside yourself using a technique I call the Multiple Perspective Advantage, or MPA. It allows you to objectify, externalize, and distance yourself from a situation to provide a better perspective, which can help you assess your own feelings and emotions when it comes to the regret you are facing and find the courage to move forward.

A great way to practice this is to use two chairs, where you move from one to the other, as if you were a friend or therapist advising yourself. Say the "regret" in one chair, then move to the other chair and "advise" yourself, discussing how you could see this situation differently. If you don't have two chairs, you can visualize this or just move from one spot to another—whatever works for you.

Another helpful way to manage your regret in the moment by standing outside of yourself is by using what Edward de Bono called the "six thinking hats" technique, which involves looking at a problem from six different perspectives.[11] This can help you look at the situation from multiple points of view, which not only helps you stand outside of your own emotional response but also gives you a chance to calm down your brain and body.

Black hat: Use a negative perspective. What do you regret? Why does it feel so bleak?

Blue hat: Think broadly. What is the best overall solution to this regret?

Green hat: Think creatively. What are some alternative ways of viewing this regret?

Red hat: Look at the situation emotionally. What do your feelings tell you, and what are they doing to you? What are some better emotions you need to move forward today?

White hat: Look at the situation objectively. What are the facts?

Yellow hat: Use a positive perspective. How can you make this regret work for you and not against you?

To download the table from this chapter, visit helpinahurrybook.com/resources

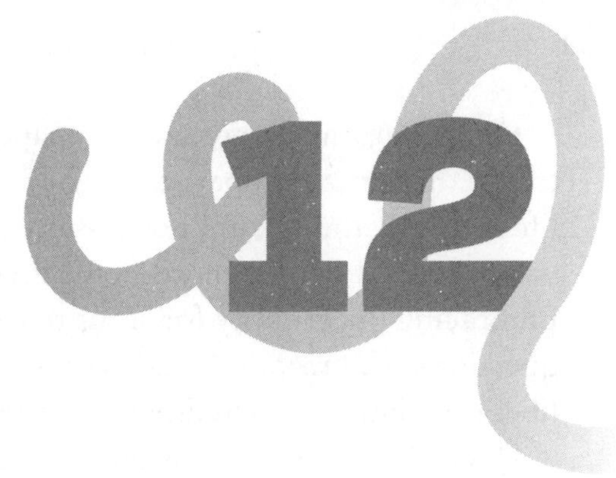

Help, I Don't Know What the Heck Is Happening!

When we are going through a tough time, it's natural to want to find the easiest route out of it. It's also natural to want to find some level of control when everything seems like it is falling apart. We want to know what works, why something happened, or why someone did something—a formula that tells us what to *do* and takes all the ambiguity out of what has happened or is happening to us. We want something "real," something "certain," that guarantees that if we do *x*, *y* will happen and things will get better.

Yet, as is so often the case in life, the one thing we can be certain of is the uncertain. So much is either out of our control or unknown. One of the strangest, and perhaps ironic, elements of healing is the fact that we often find solutions and move forward when we embrace this ambiguity and vagueness; when we accept that we cannot control what happens to us but can control how we choose to react to it.

Of course, this sounds great on paper. Who wouldn't want to put that on a bumper sticker or fridge magnet? But real life is messy, and the unknown is often terrifying. What are we supposed to do when we are staring right into that abyss? Embracing uncertainty forces us to examine, confront, ask questions of, face, and deal with our fears, which can be liberating but also incredibly overwhelming.

Uncertainty can also often make us feel like our safety and security are at risk. Things seem so completely out of our control that it is almost hopeless. What can we do if we don't even know what the heck is happening? This is almost like a virus, something that feels like it is jeopardizing our survival and ramping up our internal fight-or-flight instinct, especially if past traumas have made us afraid of the mysterious. It's so natural for our normal human mind to search desperately for a reason, an explanation—anything to help rationalize the frightening or terrible uncertainty caused by something that has happened.

In many cases, uncertainty is triggering because society makes us feel that if we don't have our stuff together, then it's all our fault. *Externally*, we feel pressure to have our life in order all the time. The uncertainty of sickness is a good example of this: It is often seen or imagined as a sign of moral, ethical, or spiritual weakness.

Internally, uncertainty can make us feel like our head is a mess. Our psychoneurobiology works well on balance and coherence, so when we are afraid of the unknown, we experience this disorder holistically in a tangible, powerful, and real way throughout our mind, brain, and body. It is not just all "in our heads."

It is not uncommon for us to react to uncertainty by suppressing our fears of the unknown. Say, for example, you are dealing with a mysterious illness and know you must go through a series of uncomfortable diagnostic and treatment processes that feel like they will provide no answer. You may pretend that nothing is wrong and keep super busy to avoid going through the testing process or do as little as possible—until your body gets the better of you and these tests become unavoidable. You are practicing suppressing what you are dealing with and, before you know it, three weeks have passed, then six weeks, then nine weeks, and you have developed a habit of suppressing your fear of the unknown, which is only making you feel worse mentally and physically, while the unknown doesn't go away.

It is normal to think that uncertainty sucks. It can be scary and awful to not feel in control. But if we want to move forward in life, we need to give ourselves permission to face the darkness and mystery of uncertainty—to take that first step. This takes time, but it is a skill that will serve us well, as the unknown is unavoidable. We either learn to face uncertainty, or we let the unknown push and pull us in any direction it takes.

Although it may not seem like it, it is possible to become more comfortable with uncertainty and use it to your advantage. In the way that nausea, sweating, and so on are ways the body frees itself from toxic matter, embracing your mental pain and accepting the uncertainty that comes along with it can help you free yourself from a toxic experience, whether it's a negative habit you have developed or a trauma you have experienced.

Here are some useful, quick tips to help you do this in your life when things seem so uncertain or when you don't know what is happening or will happen in the moment.

1. Practice Standing Outside Yourself

A technique I mentioned in the previous chapter, the MPA (Multiple Perspective Advantage) can teach you to objectify, externalize, and distance yourself from a situation to provide a better perspective. This can help you assess your own feelings and emotions when it comes to the uncertainty you are facing and find the courage to move forward.

The MPA can be used anytime you feel you can't see the path ahead—when those moments feel so overwhelming that you almost feel paralyzed. Your psychoneurobiological network is designed to respond to the MPA by firing up the frontal lobe with lots of gamma waves, which helps you gain clarity and insight into a challenging situation and move forward in a creative and objective way. This, in turn, can help reduce both the physical and mental discomfort of uncertainty by giving you back some control over the situation even as you face the unknown.

Pretend you are talking to yourself as if you were speaking to a friend. You can do this in front of a mirror, using two chairs where you swap from one to another as you talk to your "friend," or in whatever way works for you. Ask the other version of you a lot of "why" questions and then write down your reflections to help organize your thinking. You can even use your imagination and view this like a movie scene!

Here are some simple questions to ask yourself as you do this, which will help make the physical pain of uncertainty more manageable as you think about and answer them:

- What do I fear? Why?
- Why do things feel so uncertain? What is the unknown in this situation? (Try to be as specific as possible.)
- Is this something I can control or had control over?
- If not, what can I do about this to gain some sense of control in my life? What does this mean for how

I choose to react right now? (Help "you" work it out by giving yourself advice.)

As you do this, think of the situation like an academic or sports challenge: Tell yourself you've got this! Remind yourself of times you have succeeded in the past to encourage you to keep on keeping on. Indeed, when you are struggling to be present and stay in the moment or struggling to be energized, looking at the past helps you see how far you have come and helps you regain your sense of peace and find hope in the midst of the chaos of life.

The more this becomes a habit, the more you will be able to let go of just focusing on the negative (i.e., always thinking *This will end badly*) and understand that things may work out better this time. You will also be able to change and adapt to your circumstances, shifting your coping strategies and harnessing what you need most to get through what you are facing.

But remember to tell yourself that it is okay to struggle, because that is how you will learn and grow. As you work through this exercise, also make space for the uncomfortable. Remind yourself that there will be difficult days, and that this is *okay* and a normal part of life. Don't feel guilty for having normal reactions to life's ups and downs, which will only compound your feelings of overwhelm and hopelessness.

2. Have a Game Plan to Develop Mental Agility

If you start feeling any kind of fear of the unknown, say, "I will do *x* and *y*." This is like taking a test; you don't know what is going to be asked, but if you study broadly enough with good mastery, you will be prepared for all eventualities.

Because so much in life is unknown, you need to plan for different outcomes. You can do this by actively looking for small "uncertainties" to build up your tolerance, gradually exposing yourself to the unknown and unplanned on purpose. For example, you could randomly reach out to that friend you haven't seen in a while, choose at the last minute to go to a different restaurant, or wake up and decide to try a different morning routine that day.

You can also use visualization techniques to do this, like imagining you are in a movie scene. Envisage the best- and worst-case scenarios and then plan how you would deal with them so that if they do happen, you are not thrown off guard. For example, maybe you have been dealing with a difficult family member who makes you feel constantly on edge because you are unsure how they are going to behave at a family gathering. You could visualize all the past occasions you interacted with this family member and how you managed those. Then, imagine some different scenarios that could happen and visualize how you see yourself managing those based on your past successes with this person and on new ways you have planned to respond (say, for instance, you want to set more boundaries with this person). So you are essentially visualizing a predictable scenario, then imagining yourself handling it in various ways.

This is different from positive thinking. You don't pretend that everything will be all right, and you have a plan for when or if things go wrong. This mindset sees and plans for multiple possibilities, good and bad, in any given situation, making sure you are prepared for a challenge and don't just react impulsively to the unknown. Listing these out on paper, or even on your phone or device, can be really helpful. The more prepared you are, the less power the unknown will have over you.

Here's how to do this step-by-step:

- Recall by visualizing in as much detail as possible, as though you are in a movie scene, your past successes in dealing with uncertainty.
- Focus on the fact that you've overcome stressful events in the past. Do this with compassion; remember to treat yourself as you would a friend going through a similar issue.
- Now, visualize what you did during that event that was helpful and what you might like to do differently next time. Write this down.
- Next, visualize yourself accepting the reality of the uncertainty in this present moment. This may sound counterintuitive, but acceptance, not resignation, is about meeting life where it is in the moment and choosing to move forward from there. Here's a good quote by mathematician John Allen Paulos to help you with this: "Uncertainty is the only certainty there is."[1]
- Now, shift from asking why to *how*. Visualize yourself answering this in as many ways as possible. For example, instead of "Why is this happening to me?" try "How can I change this situation?"

3. Expect Good Things

Even though life can be uncertain, expecting good things to come out of the unknown increases the chance that these good things will happen, because your expectations are built into the structure of your brain, affecting how you see and perceive what goes on around you.

I call this the *expectancy mindset*. You plan for the best and the worst, as mentioned above, but you hope for the best. Due to the mind-body connection, this expectancy produces real, neurophysiological outcomes in your brain and body. Doing this strengthens your psychoneurobiology, increasing the chance that what you hope will happen actually happens. When you learn to expect good things, good things often start to happen, such as better mental and physical fitness and performance.

This is not just positive thinking. You hope for the best, but you also think about the worst thing that could happen, then immediately also consider how you could transform this into something beneficial and choose to focus your attention on that.

The best way to do this is to reframe how you see what happened if the worst did come about. How can you see this as a learning opportunity? How will it help you grow? For example, you can focus on things like how this will improve your character and what you can learn, even if the worst does come about and even if the only thing you will learn is what not to do in the future, which is still incredibly helpful information.

Reconceptualizing in this way is very effective because it is a self-regulated process that engages the whole brain and body and helps change your thinking in tangible ways (through the process of neuroplasticity). As you reconceptualize or reframe something, you will feel like you are getting control of it, which makes your neurophysiology work for you and not against you, preparing you for the future regardless of what actually happens.

This is intensely satisfying because it is a creative process, moving you out of a negative spiral, which in turn makes you feel mentally and physically stronger, more capable, and in control. As a result, you are less thrown by the inevitable ups and downs of life, and you experience greater inner peace and less turmoil when facing the unknown. And, once you have mastered this one thing, it's so much easier to apply it to all your issues—it is the gift that keeps on giving.

Indeed, the more you practice this, especially when the uncertainty you are facing is more manageable or when you have just gotten through a difficult period of uncertainty, the more this is going to help you when things really feel hopeless.

Below is a table you can use to help you do this. The last part of the table is for you to fill out either at another time or if you are thinking about a past situation or experience and doing a type of mental autopsy of what happened.

For example, say you have a big project due at work, and this will determine your future at the company. You can plan and do all the work, but there are many factors outside of your control that are stressing you out, making you feel ill, affecting your sleep, and impacting your mental clarity. This, in turn, is making you feel worse and compounding your fears that you will not succeed, even though the stakes are so high.

Someone recommends you take some time to rest, calm down, and remind yourself of times you succeeded in the past. You do this but decide to take it further. You write down what is making you feel so afraid. Then you write down your plan: what you will do if things go well, and what you will do if things go badly. If the project is rejected or criticized, you won't lose your job, but that promotion you have been hoping for may be in jeopardy. You will then think of other ways you can make yourself invaluable to the company and how you can show management what you are currently contributing and what you hope to contribute in the future. You realize this may take longer than expected, but you will not give up. You know you have put in the work, and that is the most important factor—the other factors are out of your control, so there is no point worrying about them. The key thing is that you have a plan if things go badly.

However, you also have a plan if things go well, and you are choosing to focus on this too. When you find yourself slipping into that negative thought spiral, you remind yourself of your expectations and of how this experience is strengthening your mind, body, and brain, making it more likely that what you hope for will happen *and* making it more likely that even if the worst happens, you've got this! You can make this situation work for you and not against you. You do have control even when things feel so out of your control.

Below is an example of how this can look. You can also write it down in another way that works for you or download this table with spaces to work into using the QR code at the end of the chapter.

Using My Expectancy Mindset

The uncertainty	My plan	My expectations	What happened, and how I made this work for me

The uncertainty	My plan	My expectations	What happened, and how I made this work for me

4. Build Your Brain

Working on your mental fitness by building your brain will help you be more open to change because it increases your cognitive flexibility, resilience, and ability to deal with a challenge. It also helps reduce the discomfort of uncertainty by expanding your knowledge base. You are less likely to find things uncertain if you know more about humanity and the world around you.

Brain-building is, essentially, the process of *using your mind* to build or "feed" your brain on a regular basis, just like you need to eat every day to nourish your body. It's the process of feeding the brain regularly with new and challenging information (the "healthy food") that is then "well digested," or *deeply understood*.

The actual process of brain-building is incredibly rapid. Genes are activated within a few minutes, and a single neuron can gain thousands of new dendritic branches in a very short time. This is one of the first things I would train my patients to do when I was in private practice. As I mentioned above, it's a powerful tool; my early research showed up to 75 percent improvement in academic, cognitive, social, emotional, and intellectual function when people were taught how to build their brain and harness deep, intellectual thought.[2]

When you build your brain, you build your resilience and your intelligence. This changes the way energy flows through the brain, optimizing its function and cognitive flexibility. Brain-building also uses the thousands of new baby nerve cells that are born when you wake up each morning, called *neurogenesis*. If you don't use these baby nerve cells and don't brain-build, toxic waste can build up in the brain that may affect your mood and sleep. It can also lower the resilience of the brain, increasing your vulnerability to the unknown.

So, every day, take the time to build your brain: Listen to podcasts, read books (fiction or nonfiction) and/or the news, learn a language, or whatever strikes your fancy. Try new things, especially something that challenges you. At first it may be scary, but, over time, the scary feeling of being a "novice" will subside. Like exercise, the more you do this, the stronger you will get; the more you live a life of welcoming the unknown in this small but effective way, the less of a threat it becomes in your life.

Getting out of your comfort zone is also a great way to build your brain by exposing yourself to new experiences, new people, new ideas, and new ways of living. Travel can take many forms—you don't just have to visit a foreign country to train yourself to embrace the unknown and the uncertain and expand your worldview. Even a short road trip can teach you a lot about how to manage how you feel in new and unfamiliar situations, with the added bonus of learning something and building your brain.

5. Have a Support System in Place

Having someone you trust to confide in and ask for advice is so important if you are going through a period of uncertainty. Not only does this help you not feel alone and threatened but it also can provide perspective, and it may help you make a plan of action to deal with the uncertainty.

This person could be a therapist, counselor, friend, or family member you trust and whom you feel safe with. By talking about what you fear, you externalize it, which makes it easier to deal with because it is no longer hidden.

We all, to some degree, fear uncertainty and the unknown; this is a part of being human. Don't be ashamed to share your fears with those you trust. More than likely, they will be able not only to give you a different perspective to help you manage your uncertainty but to relate to you and share their own similar experiences, which will make you feel less alone.

6. Make Your Mental Self-Care a Priority

Reading fiction, having fun, taking time out, exercising, eating well, doing something creative each day, sleeping more, daydreaming more, meditating, or whatever helps you relax and brings you joy are, strangely enough, great ways to help prepare for the unknown. Making sure to make time for you, however that looks, will help build up your mental toughness and stress resilience.

This is kind of like an insurance policy: You invest in the good times so that you can handle the bad times. Or, to put it another way, this is similar to what athletes do to prepare for a challenge like a competition. You are training your mind and brain so that it is less likely to be thrown by the inevitable unknowns in life.

The more you make mental self-care a priority in your life, the more you are ready for whatever comes your way. This is not selfish or self-centered. If you don't take care of you in the now, which includes embracing moments of rest and joy, then you won't be much help to yourself or even others in the future.

To download the table from this chapter, visit helpinahurrybook.com/resources

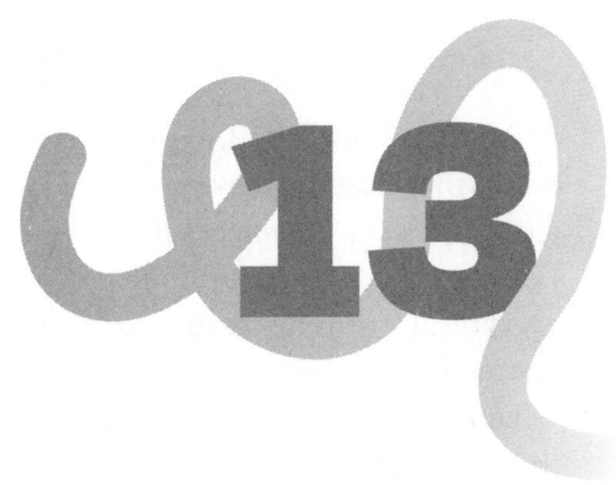

Help, My Past Is Haunting Me!

Childhood trauma is a major topic of discussion these days, and for good reason. What we experience when we are young and just starting to find our place in the world can have a major impact on our mental, emotional, and physical health in adulthood. As children, we are so vulnerable, and our understanding of the world and ourselves is influenced by the adults around us and the events we experience.

Research on this topic shows us just how important adverse childhood events are when it comes to our health. One of the most famous points of research in this area is the early '90s landmark study of over seventeen thousand individuals that asked them about negative experiences in childhood and their current physical and mental health.[1] This study found that when children are exposed to toxic stress hormones like cortisol and adrenaline, this can have a dramatic impact on their minds, brains, and bodies.[2] This study later became known as the Adverse Childhood Experiences or ACEs study.[3]

Adverse childhood experiences (ACEs) are traumatic events that children may be exposed to that include abuse, neglect, domestic violence, substance misuse, or mental illness. Long-term exposure to childhood trauma has been linked to everything from heart disease and diabetes to alcoholism, depression, and suicide.[4]

Unfortunately, this is a global problem. Research shows that around 61.5 percent of adults and 48 percent of children have been exposed to ACEs.[5] The scope and impact are things we all need to be aware of so that more and more people can get the help they need to heal and recover.[6]

While there is no denying the reality and impact of adverse childhood experiences on our mental and physical health, just focusing on the negative alone, or the bad that happened to us, may actually slow down the process of our healing. Research on the mind-brain-body network shows that an overly negative focus can distort our perceptions and potentially hamstring our ability to work through what we have gone through in a way that doesn't keep us trapped in the past.[7]

The mind-brain-body network is all about balance—and restoring balance when it is upset. Focusing only on the negative will add to an already overloaded amount of toxic stress brought on by the adverse experience. This is why it is important that, while we do the work to find the root causes of our distress and process and reconceptualize what has happened to us, we also make sure we have *positive* checkpoints in place on our healing journey. Otherwise we risk getting stuck in a cycle of pain and victimhood.

In fact, there is exciting research that shows that positive childhood experiences (PCEs) can help buffer against the negative health effects caused by exposure to ACEs.[8] PCEs can also promote healing and recovery through activating our resilience.[9] This shows that all of a child's experiences—positive and negative—matter, so we shouldn't just consider the bad that has happened to us but also the good. *All* these experiences affect our mental and emotional health as adults.

Some research even shows that people with some exposure to ACEs, if they reported three to five positive childhood experiences, had 50 percent lower odds of adulthood depression or poor mental health. Those who reported six to seven PCEs had a 72 percent lower chance of adult mental health challenges.[10] These findings demonstrate that positive childhood experiences can have a cumulative effect on lifelong mental health outcomes and play an important role in our healing.

Constantly focusing on the negative can saturate our mindsets to the point where we feel we don't have a choice because everything feels so hopeless. It can make us feel fragile, broken, and worthless when everything seems so bleak. And if we are constantly surrounded by messages that tell us how adverse childhood experiences equate to mental and physical problems in adulthood, without giving us much hope to go on in the opposite direction, this may inadvertently send the message of "What's the point of even trying if I am so damaged anyway?" Awareness of an issue is not enough and can often make things seem so much worse.

We also have to be careful of conflating adversity with trauma, as not all hardship is bad.[11] This perspective, seeing all "bad" as trauma, can quickly suck the joy out of every moment. As journalist Gary Walsh notes,

> While abuse and neglect should always be considered fundamentally wrong, traumatic and preventable, the same cannot always be said for adversity. Everyone will experience adversity at some point and there is often strength and hope to be

found in it. Our responses to adversity can nurture resilience and loving relationships while also defining our identities.[12]

Relying on our feelings alone can also be confusing. When we are processing a toxic emotion, it's very normal to feel "under the weather," even though we have to face these uncomfortable emotions in order to heal. If not managed, these feelings can spread like a virus, shaping all our thoughts and snowballing into a big, negative mindset that can influence how we feel and approach the rest of the day, week, month, year . . . until it is faced, processed, and reconceptualized. Thoughts can quickly become distorted if we just focus on the negative. Yes, it is important to address past traumas and work through them, but the more we ruminate on them, the more power they will have over our life and the less hope we will have for the future. It's all about balance!

This is why the research on PCEs is so exciting. Understanding how they interact with adverse experiences to help mitigate the effects of ACEs is extremely hopeful and really highlights the plasticity of the mind-brain-body network. We always need to remind ourselves that the brain can change and heal, as the PCEs research suggests. Finding something good, even the smallest thing, can help mitigate the enormous impact unresolved childhood experiences may have had on us or that we may be passing on to our own children.[13]

We need to try to avoid looking at our childhood as binary "either/or," or simply good or bad. Rather, a healthier approach is to see the past as "both/and." Both good and bad things have happened to us, and we need to focus on the full, complex picture if we want to find healing. Barring obvious and unacceptable traumatic experiences, most children grow up with some negative impact from the parenting they received because parents are only human. Many parents do the best they can in the moment and are struggling with the effects of their own upbringing.

Of course, we have to work on the impact of what we experienced growing up, but, at the same time, in many cases we need to hold room for compassion toward our parents and guardians, recognizing the challenges they, too, faced. For example, in my own life, my father was emotionally absent, even though he always worked hard to provide for our physical needs. Part of my journey as both a child and a parent was understanding that his behavior stemmed from his own experiences: My father was put into boarding school at age four and had little nurturing or emotional care from his own parents for years. I do not excuse his lack of emotional support or my own needs as a child for that care and comfort, but I do recognize that, to a degree, he did what he knew and what he thought made him a good enough father. I honor his memory in the best way I know how: by acknowledging that he was human, imperfect, and still made me smile and gave me some of my most treasured memories.

When we face our past, the key thing to remember is that it is not a zero-sum game and focusing on the negative alone or ignoring the bad that happened to us will not help us heal or move forward in life. Indeed, either extreme can keep us trapped, impacting not only our present but also our future, making us more vulnerable to mental and physical ill-health.

As a mental health professional and advocate, I am more than aware of how adverse experiences can affect us. My work, research, and mental health platform are all about helping people deconstruct and reconstruct these experiences to change how they play out into the future. Partly this means facing the bad and terrible but not in a way that ends up giving these things more power over us. I want to see people free to live their best lives, and I know this is possible. There is so much hope, even if the healing journey is a long and hard one.

This is why I emphasize balancing the good, bad, and ugly of our pasts, which will help us tap into the incredible well of resilience we have as human beings by asking for help, developing trusting relationships, forming a positive attitude, listening to our feelings, and learning how to embrace, process, and reconceptualize past traumas. When we learn how to do this, we can feel empowered to start rewriting our own story as we find true and lasting healing and joy in life.

This is something I want for everyone, and it starts in the small moments—those everyday struggles we all face that have the power to keep us stuck in negative patterns and habits if we don't learn how to manage them. Below are two "help in a hurry" tips to get you through these moments, shift your focus from the negative alone, and remind you that life is more than just any ACEs in your past.

These steps are not designed to heal all your trauma, which takes time and deliberate effort and often requires a lot of professional and personal support. Rather, they are there to assist you in the moment when you are alone and find yourself struggling with feelings of overwhelm, despondency, and hopelessness—those moments when the past is so crippling that you are not even sure where to turn or what to do.

1. Balance Your ACEs and PCEs

This first tip is more of a self-evaluation exercise to see if you do, perhaps, have any potential ACEs that need attention, which you can then balance with your PCEs so you do not get stuck just focusing on the negative, which will affect your ability to heal, as mentioned above.

Finding My Balance

Question	Answer
Was my childhood all bad? (Describe.)	
Can I recall and describe any positive experiences?	
Have I been influenced by the vast amount of exposure to adversity and/or traumatic childhood experiences? How?	
Have I balanced the good with the bad, or have I gotten sucked into the wrong direction by focusing only on the negative?	
Can I find the balance between understanding adversity in my childhood and how this has impacted me and the challenges my own parents dealt with?	

Completing this first exercise will take a little time to do and is more proactive in nature. It is designed to help you to (1) evaluate whether you are in a negative state of mind from unmanaged adverse childhood experiences and (2) balance this with your more positive experiences of childhood.

The second tip is something quick you can do in the moment to help you get out of a trauma spiral, but it will be more effective if you have done this self-evaluation when you have more time on your hands.

However, you are welcome to skip this if you feel you are not ready, or do it with a therapist, counselor, or friend if you feel it could be triggering. Tip 2, below, is very helpful and works really well for any negative mindset, not just for dealing with past traumas.

2. Practice the 3:1 Thought Ratio

Although we all definitely need to work on what we experienced growing up, at the same time we need to leave room for the positive, and a great way to do this is what I call the "3:1 thought ratio." This is one technique I often use to balance myself, and I find it extremely helpful when things seem overwhelming. All it involves is intentionally focusing on the positive to balance out the negative in a 3:1 ratio. This can be used for any negative situation, not just for ACEs.

For every negative thought that comes to mind, along with its emotions, behaviors, and perspectives, counter it with three positive thoughts. This will help to maintain a balance in energy (quantum) waves in the brain so you can think clearly, build your resilience, and rewire your thought patterns.

So, each time you have a negative thought, don't suppress it but rather use it as a prompt to think of three positive childhood experiences. This doesn't mean you are ignoring what has happened to you; rather, you are maintaining the balance of your mind, brain, and body so that you can heal what has happened to you rather than remaining trapped in the past.

You are essentially using the negative thought as a habit loop trigger to help you recognize what to change *while* "padding" or mitigating the effects this negative event has on your overall well-being. This is not swapping the negative for the positive. It is using the positive to help yourself face and overcome the negative.

Why a 3:1 ratio? Research by Dr. Barbara Fredrickson has indicated that there's a tipping point of at least three to one in terms of positivity to negativity to keep the brain and body in balance.[14] Toxic emotional states can cause too much high beta and high gamma energy, which make us feel awful and cause the energy in the brain to swish violently about like a tsunami, which we see as red spots, or foci, on the head maps of the qEEG (which measures the energy frequencies in the brain).[15] To rebalance this energy, the nonconscious mind grabs our attention through emotional and physical warning signals to tell us to fix it, and that fix requires managing what we focus on.

As you work through this exercise, it is important to remember that a negative thought or emotion isn't necessarily toxic. Sometimes thinking about the worst-case scenario for a limited time period can help us prepare for the unknown so that we feel more in control, and it can also help us be more creative, adaptable, and realistic when we are faced with the ups and downs of life.

I would also recommend setting a time limit for how long you spend focusing on the negative. Under five minutes is what I would usually tell my patients when I was practicing.

Below is a table of examples to get you started. You can use a table like this to help you list your thoughts in a 3:1 ratio, which you can also download using the QR code at the end of the chapter, or you can note them down in another format or say them out loud—whatever works for you!

3:1 Ratio Examples	
My dad was physically and emotionally distant.	• My dad was always there when I needed him, even if he was emotionally distant at times. • My dad would often smile at me when he dropped me off at school. • My dad showed how proud he was of me when I did something well by wiping small tears from his eyes with a smile.
My parents argued a lot.	• My parents showed a lot of love for each other as well. • My big sister would always take me into her room and explain what was happening, and then we would watch a movie or read a funny book together. • My parents always used to check in on me after an argument and would tuck me into bed before I went to sleep every night. This is how they showed they cared.
As a child, I felt like my family had to avoid talking about "deep" or "hard" topics.	• My family had amazing holidays when I was growing up. • Every Sunday, my family had a special lunch where friends and extended family were invited, and it was such a happy time. • i have spoken more with my family as I have gotten older, which has helped me process a lot of what happened in the past and improved my relationship with my parents.

To download the tables from this chapter, visit helpinahurrybook .com/resources

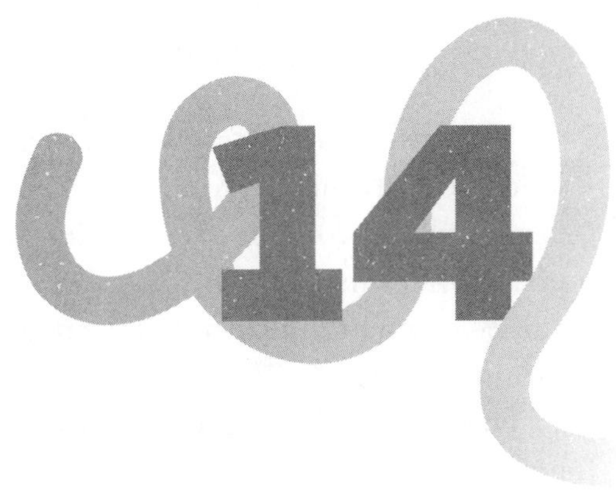

Help, I'm a People Pleaser!

It is perfectly natural to want people to like us—no one wakes up wanting to be shunned or hated. The desire to engage with and please others is common, and it is not a cause for concern in small amounts. We are social beings, and community plays a major role in our mental and physical well-being.

But when does this natural longing turn us into people pleasers? When does our desire to be loved turn toxic and make us do and say things that are not true to who we are or who we want to be?

It is important to note that there is a difference between a people pleaser and a peacemaker. A peacemaker wants to restore balance and reach a resolution and tries to see the issue from all sides in a rational and objective way. This person has a desire to help others; consequently, they will sometimes be willing to say the truth even if it hurts and even if the people involved do not want to face reality.

A people pleaser, however, is more self-focused and afraid of criticism. This person tends to be hypersensitive to uncertainty and conflict and feels a strong urge to please others. As a result, they will be more willing to sacrifice their values or mental health and even change their personality around others.

This creates a toxic feedback loop: A people pleaser seeks approval because of their low self-confidence, which further lowers the value they place on themselves and will weaken their resolve to stand up to people in the future. This can be quite dangerous; sometimes others who pick up on this desire to please can take advantage of the person in question, making them say and do things that go against their integrity.

However, low self-confidence is not the only factor that can lead to people-pleasing. Someone may be scared to confront a person because of what they may say or do and how they react in general. This often happens when we have a loved one who is battling with mental health issues, addictions, or narcissistic type personality issues. In these situations, pleasing a person is often associated with a strong desire to keep that person in a safe place, but in doing so, our own mental health ends up being compromised. If this is happening in your life, it's important to get support and guidance from a professional or someone you trust in addition to applying the ideas and tips presented in this chapter, as these conflicts can quickly spiral and result in a lot of pain and anxiety.

When it comes to people-pleasing in general, it is important to ask *why* we tend to be so averse to conflict. Why do we not like being not liked, even to the point of going against what we believe or our own values? The answer lies largely in our human nature, which is the core fabric of our mind-brain-body network: We are designed for deep, meaningful connections, as mentioned earlier. Not being liked goes against our social nature; we cannot understand it, which is not only painful but also makes us feel unsure about ourselves.

Subsequently, we look for ways to reduce this uncertainty and pain by making ourselves less vulnerable. In other words, we look for ways to pander to people to get them to like and accept us into their "group." So being a people pleaser is a kind of survival instinct—we do it partly to avoid facing and dealing with our self-confidence problems, which is a painful process, and partly because we really need people to like us.

Ultimately, people-pleasing is like any behavior: In moderation, it can actually be a good thing. We want to be nice and helpful to others, so a little "pleasing" can go a long way in making another person feel special—as long as it's done authentically, with kindness, and without compromising our own values or sense of self. But pleasing others can quickly spiral out of control and become a negative habit, especially when we are in a vulnerable position in life or dealing with a lot of past pain and trauma. Here are some key signs associated with people-pleasing:

- finding it hard to say no
- regularly taking on extra work, even if you don't have the time
- overcommitting to plans, responsibilities, or projects
- saying you are fine when you aren't
- avoiding disagreeing with people
- holding back your honest opinion
- going along with things you are not happy about just to avoid upsetting someone
- feeling pressure to be friendly and nice

- feeling like your own wants or needs don't matter in comparison to others'
- feeling that other people take advantage of you

When we are focused on pleasing people, we can end up sacrificing our self-identity, our morals and values, and our mental health. This creates feelings of resentment toward the people we are trying to impress or keep happy, and we can quickly develop a sense of victimization as we lose more and more of our own authenticity, which in turn can end up creating a toxic feedback loop.

The more we act in this manner, the stronger this neural pathway becomes in the brain, and we can end up becoming addicted to pleasing people despite how it makes us feel. We get a temporary "high" as we make someone else happy, and we keep doing it to get that same high again and again. This addictive behavior can create disorder in the mind-brain-body network, which can be very disruptive and affect our health and well-being.

It also can become a self-fulfilling prophecy. If we feel that people are not giving us the feedback or responses we need, we tend to try to please them even more, which further decreases our sense of self and our confidence.

People-pleasing takes away the opportunity for us to define our own path, which will only add to our internal frustration. We are essentially working against who we are. This sense of frustration will be compounded by the fact that the relationships we form and grow are unstable: People are only attracted to us because we have changed ourselves to please them, which is not sustainable in the long run. Eventually, such relationships will fail, leaving us feeling isolated and drained, which will further impact our mental health, and we will be less motivated to make an effort to connect with other people.

People-pleasing is a type of cognitive dissonance. When we lie to ourselves and are not true to who we are and what we want, we can experience an internal "war"—what we say and do is not in agreement with what we are thinking about or what we value. This can impact both our mental and physical health. A lack of mental congruence drains our energy, causing toxic stress and affecting the way information is processed and memory is built, which sets us up for neurochemical chaos in the brain and body.

Needless to say, getting trapped in a people-pleasing cycle is not fun. It can be incredibly disruptive to your day-to-day life, making it hard to even make simple decisions or know what to do. If this rings a bell, below are several strategies you can practice to take back control in the moment and start redefining who you are and what you want in life.

1. Be Honest with Yourself

I know this sounds obvious and a little clichéd, but when you are stuck in a habit of people-pleasing, being honest with yourself really is the first and most important step you can take to break the cycle. You must first acknowledge that you need to change, admit you have a problem, and become aware of your thoughts and actions around people before you can truly change and heal.

After you have taken this first, difficult step, practice observing how you behave over a period of time and what other people may say or have said to you about your behavior. Be very kind and compassionate toward yourself while you do this. Constantly remind yourself that this isn't who you are but rather who you have become and that you can "unbecome" it.

These are painful and uncomfortable acknowledgments and observations, but do not let that get you down. Tune in to the discomfort—this will help you recognize the need to change and show you where you need to change.

To do this, I recommend tracking your people-pleasing over a week or two. Write this down in the following table, which you can also download at the QR code at the end of the chapter, or use whatever method works best for you. Doing this will help you bring clarity to the situation and organize your thinking so you know what needs to change.

My People-Pleasing Tracker

People-pleasing incident	When? Where? How often? Did someone say something to you?

People-pleasing incident	When? Where? How often? Did someone say something to you?

2. Analyze Your Behavior

If you are uncertain if people-pleasing is an issue in your life, below is a table you can fill in to see if you are showing signs of being a people pleaser. You can also use whatever system works best for you or download this table using the QR code at the end of the chapter. If you answer yes to a lot of these questions, remember you are only human and it's okay not to be okay. You can learn how not to be a people pleaser; this behavior is not set in stone.

Once you become aware of how much people-pleasing has become a habit in your life, ask yourself who, what, when, where, why, and how. Say, for example, you had a tough childhood and felt that you could never please your parents. Does your desire to have people like you stem from your relationship with your parents? Or does it come from another bad relationship?

This will help you get to the root of the issue and start working on it so it doesn't keep impacting your day-to-day life. Once you are aware of what is happening, you can start brainstorming ways to shift how you think about something and practice this in your life. Taking the example above: You acknowledge that people-pleasing is something that comes from a negative relationship, and you can then shift your focus to other, more positive relationships in your life and think about why those people value their time with you. You can list what they love about you and what you are proud of, and you can remind yourself of this every time you feel the need to compromise your values in order to be liked.

When it comes to changing a toxic habit, it is so important that your words and actions align with your thoughts, so mentally prepare yourself, practice saying no when you find yourself facing the urge to please someone, and spend more time defining and identifying what you want and who you want to be. You will never be okay with someone not liking who you are unless you practice being okay with conflict and uncertainty—and recognize that not everyone will like you, and that is perfectly okay too.

You can also do this step with a therapist, mental health professional, or someone you trust if you feel that this is triggering or upsetting you.

Am I a People Pleaser?

Question	**If yes, describe who, what, when, where, why, and how *and* how this is affecting you.**	**What can you do instead? How can you shift the way you think and act?**
Are you doing anything possible to avoid conflict, even if it means turning into an entirely different person?		
Does your self-worth depend on how others see you?		

Question	If yes, describe who, what, when, where, why, and how *and* how this is affecting you.	What can you do instead? How can you shift the way you think and act?
Do you need validation from others to feel good about yourself?		
Does your natural longing to be accepted and liked affect how you treat others and/or how you let them treat you?		
Do you do and say things that are not true to who you are or who you want to be?		
Do you go to the extreme to earn words of praise from others?		
Do you feel like you always have to say yes?		
Do you compromise your integrity to keep the peace and shun conflict?		
Do you ever feel uncomfortable with something but do it anyway?		
Do you ever feel like you have no clear identity?		
Do you feel that you lack your own vision and goals?		

3. Get to Know Yourself Again

When we fall into a pattern of people-pleasing, it is easy to lose sight of who we are and what we love. This is why, if people-pleasing is an issue in your life, you should take the time to get to know yourself again, and one of the best ways to do this is to rediscover what you love.

Some ways you can do this are:

- Think about times you were happiest or at peace and try to re-create those times. What made them special? How did they make you feel more "alive"?
- Explore! Read books on all kinds of topics to discover what interests you, listen to more podcasts, watch TV shows or documentaries that you enjoy, learn a new language or skill that excites you, take up a new hobby that you think you will like, and so on. Even if you find that something doesn't really engage you like you thought it would, just the act of being open to exploring new things and ideas that make you feel alive and more in tune with who you are and want to be will start breaking those people-pleasing chains holding you back. Just make sure you are doing these things for you and not someone else.
- Think about your ideal relationship: What does this look like? What does being happy and being yourself around another person mean to you? Visualize this and write it down. The next time you are tempted to people-please, look at what you have written and remind yourself what a healthy relationship looks like to you. Remind yourself that this is worth fighting for, even if it feels uncomfortable in the moment—which is completely normal and okay.

4. Practice Setting Boundaries

I saw a funny meme on social media the other day that had a picture of someone making a triumphant face with the caption, "people pleasers in their villain era when they set one boundary."[1] For many people pleasers, or people in general, just saying no or putting a boundary in place can make us feel like we are the "bad guy," even though it is really quite the opposite. Boundaries are not about the other person; rather, they are about us: what we are capable of and what we need to maintain or improve our mental health in that moment.

I think one of the best ways to think about boundaries is to visualize three different glasses and a small stone. One glass is tiny, like a shot glass; one glass is a tumbler; the last glass is larger, like a mason jar. In the shot glass, the little stone takes up a lot of room. In the glass tumbler, the stone takes up less room. And in the mason jar, the stone takes up hardly any room.

See this stone as an issue you are dealing with, such as a toxic person in your family, at work, or at school. This issue is very real, just like the stone is real. And, if you feel like you need a boundary, this means you feel that this person or people are invading your personal space, which can have real physical and mental repercussions. In fact, every interaction with this person adds more and more toxicity to this issue. (This is at the heart of what it means to be "triggered.") The issue gets bigger and bigger in your mind, which has a greater impact on your well-being.

A healthy way to deal with this "stone" and put up boundaries involves creating space around the issue, not permitting it to get any bigger. This allows you to gain perspective, which then enables you to get to the root cause of the issue and work on managing and reconceptualizing it.

You can't fix or change the person who is impacting you in a negative way; you can only take responsibility for your own response—that is, what you choose to do and how you choose to respond. Using the analogy of the glasses, this means moving the rock from the shot glass, where it is taking up all that space in your life and is all-consuming, to the tumbler glass, where you have more space and perspective to work on it. Then, you eventually move it to the mason jar glass, where, through healthy boundaries, it no longer defines you or your well-being. Here, you have had enough space to work on it and get to the root cause, and you are learning how to manage its impact in your life and deal with the person affecting you in a healthy way. You are working toward resolving the issue and finding the best way to move forward FOR YOU.

Here are some ways to practice this:

- When someone makes a request or asks you something, allow yourself some time to think about it rather than answering them immediately. A good rule of thumb is to give yourself at least sixty to ninety seconds to respond, practicing some deep breathing while you wait to calm down your mind, brain, and body in the moment. Of course, this is pretty easy to do over text or email, for example, but if you are talking to this person face-to-face it can be a little harder. You can say something like "I just need a minute to think about this," or excuse yourself and go to the bathroom for a few moments, especially if you feel the overwhelming urge to just say yes or agree with that person. You can then use this time to really think about what you need and if what this person is asking truly aligns with what you can do or want to do.

- If you end up agreeing to do something, put some limits in place. Set a deadline, let that person know you can only do *x* and not *y*, and so on. Don't leave the conversation or what the other person wants open-ended, or you could end up draining yourself. Also, don't let someone else dictate what you should or shouldn't do, as you know your own capabilities and needs best.
- Use space/distance to examine *why* you feel the way you do. Ask yourself questions. Why did you feel the need to people-please? Why did you show up or react in this way? How do you see yourself and this issue? What are some boundaries you can put in place to help you overcome this habit?

When you create a healthy boundary, the issue stays the same but the boundary creates the space you need to look at the issue differently, work on it, and reconceptualize it over time, thereby finding a way forward in your life. This is key! Even if the person responds negatively, you can still control *how they affect you*, which is incredibly empowering—even if setting boundaries feels challenging when you first start practicing it. Hopefully, the way you are managing yourself and are becoming less reactive will impact them, and they, too, will recognize they need to create space to work on themselves.

To download the tables from this chapter, visit helpinahurrybook .com/resources

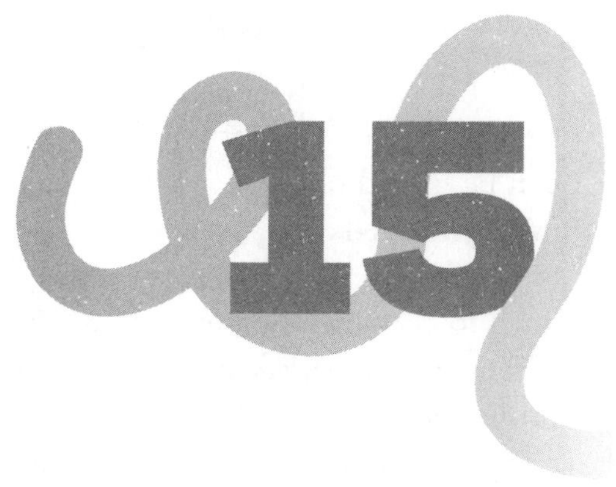

Help, My Inner Critic Won't Let Up!

Facing criticism, whether justified or not, is incredibly hard. No one wants to hear that what they have done falls short in any way. It is so easy to take someone's words, no matter how well-meaning they are, and see them as some kind of judgment on our character or self-worth.

At least, if it's coming from another person, you can still create some distance between what is said about you and how you feel about yourself. But what if the critic is you? What if you are your own worst enemy? How do you escape yourself, whom you are with 24/7?

So often in life, we are our harshest judges. We give our inner critics free rein over our thoughts, actions, and choices, letting them shape how we see ourselves and how we show up in life—and how this impacts our health and well-being.

We have all been there: listening to that voice inside our head that tells us we are not good enough or we can't do something; it constantly judges us and finds us wanting. It can be incredibly demeaning, dragging us down and keeping us trapped.

When this negative self-talk is so ingrained, it can be hard to convince ourselves that it's a bad thing—but it is! The words we speak generate energy that comes from our thoughts and impacts our mind-brain-body network.[1] They contain power and work hand in hand with our thought life because they make our thoughts "come alive," influencing the circumstances of our life. If these thoughts are positive, they can lead to amazing things. If they are negative, we can give rise to some pretty frightening, Frankenstein-like monsters in our mind.

While reflecting on our mistakes isn't a problem, and can actually be a healthy way to heal and grow, it's the hostility that can come with self-criticism that does true damage to our psyche and health. When our mind marinates in self-critical thoughts, our body releases a chaotic flood of hormones, which spikes the stress hormone cortisol and can lead to all kinds of problems if unmanaged.

There's a lot of advice out there telling us how to shut down this inner critic. But is this always helpful? What we resist persists. The more we try to suppress something, the harder it tries to sink its fingernails into us, damaging our self-confidence and ability to trust ourselves and our instincts, which can end up creating a cycle of self-blame and self-doubt.

We can't ever get rid of our personal fears and anxieties completely. In fact, in many cases they can be insightful warning signals, giving us information about ourselves and what is going on in our life. When we learn how to address and manage these feelings—when we learn how to talk back to our inner critic—we can turn a potentially toxic situation into an opportunity to learn and grow.

The key thing to remember is that we are way more capable and valuable than our inner critic says we are. The words we use as we talk to ourselves have power, but they don't have control over our reality—unless we give it to them. It is possible to learn how to work with our inner critic and manage it, while still recognizing our own importance and trusting our decisions.

Of course, this takes hard work and practice, practice, practice! As the saying goes, Rome was not built in a day. Developing a plan to really try to understand how you think, feel, and choose, as well as better understanding what you want and need as a person, can help you stay focused, make informed decisions, face your inner critic, and learn how to frame your reality with your words.

Below are some tips to help you manage your relationship with your inner critic and start practicing this in your life, especially during those moments when your self-talk feels like it is destroying you from the inside out. Remember, whatever you think about the most will grow. As you work through these tips, always pay attention to what you are focusing on the most. If you think something like *I want to believe I am good enough* while you work on the root of your negative self-talk, that *I want to believe* will eventually become *I believe*.

1. Pull Back the Curtain

When you are dealing with a lot of negative self-talk, imagine you are pulling back a curtain and seeing your inner critic in front of you as a tiny little ant "shouting" so loudly at you. This will not only create distance between you and your critic but also make it seem less overwhelming.

Next, imagine asking the ant what they're really trying to say and naming it. This may sound odd, but this simple act helps reduce the negative energy associated with this ant, and the ridiculousness of naming it can help defuse the tenseness of the situation in the moment so that you feel less stressed and overwhelmed.

2. See Your Self-Talk as a Protective Mechanism

It is natural for us to experience fear and self-blame, especially if we have been in situations in the past that have put us under tremendous stress. Remind yourself of this when you start to hear that inner voice. Acknowledge the fear—be graceful and compassionate toward your past self for looking out for you. Then, remind yourself that you are no longer in that same position and no longer have to fear that specific experience. Your past and present, although connected, are not the same. Keep telling yourself this for as long as you need to, while breathing deeply to help calm down your mind, brain, and body in the moment.

3. Don't Just Try to Silence the Voice—Question It!

If we are completely honest, we cannot always control our inner critic. The harder we try to corral these thoughts, the more stress we can experience, which can end up making the situation worse. We may feel like we are failing ourselves if the thoughts don't just "go away."

A better strategy is to question your thoughts instead of suppressing them, as I mentioned above. If your inner critic is telling you that you will fail at something, for example, question *why* it is saying that. Try to find the evidence behind the thought—become a "thought detective."

Next, try to find reasons you won't fail. Focus on the successes you have had in the past, not just your failures.

Remember the times you overcame a challenge and celebrate them. For example, change a statement like "I am not good enough" or "I'm stupid" into "I am smart—look at my achievements so far! Just because this didn't work out doesn't mean other things won't. I have already seen this in my life when . . ."

As you do this, really think about what your inner critic is trying to tell you. What is it signaling to you in your life? Below is a helpful table you can use to do this, which you can also download using the QR code at the end of the chapter. If you want, you can work through this with a therapist, professional, or someone you trust if this is something you really struggle with and you find you need more perspective to work through it.

My Inner Critic

Question	**Answer**	**What is this pointing to?**	**How can you reframe this?**
How would you describe your life?			
Do you struggle with negative self-talk?			
What words do you use to describe yourself and your life experiences?			
How would you describe yourself to someone who doesn't know you?			

(continued)

Question	Answer	What is this pointing to?	How can you reframe this?
What words do you typically use to describe your personality traits?			
How do you talk about your strengths, achievements, and successes?			
Are there any words or phrases you tend to use when discussing your weaknesses or challenges?			
What do you think others perceive about you based on the words you use to describe yourself?			
Do you notice any patterns or themes in the words you use to describe yourself?			
How do you think your self-descriptions impact your interactions with others?			
Are there any words or labels you've adopted from others to describe yourself?			
How do you feel when you hear someone else use certain words to describe you?			

Write down what you have observed about the words you use to describe yourself and frame your reality. You can do this over a period of several days. As you work through these questions, try to think deeply about how these words affect your reality and how you can change them to shift your self-talk and perspective.

The last part of the table can be challenging to work through, so here are some helpful questions you can ask yourself as you go:

- Are the things I say to myself based on facts or assumptions?
- What evidence do I have to support or refute these allegations?
- Am I being fair?
- How can I practice more self-compassion and kindness toward myself?
- Would I say these things to a loved one or friend in a similar situation?
- What alternative perspectives could I consider?
- Are there any underlying beliefs or past experiences influencing my self-talk?
- How might I reframe this criticism in a more constructive or empowering way?
- What positive qualities or achievements am I overlooking?
- What small steps can I take to challenge and gradually change this critical inner voice?

This may seem like a lot at first, but this is a really helpful exercise when it comes to examining and confronting your inner critic. You're essentially engaging in a mental autopsy, which, remember, is where you analyze your thoughts and feelings and act as your own detective to identify patterns, triggers, and activators so you can change them. As you work through these questions, remind yourself that this is an ongoing process that requires practice, patience, self-compassion, and change! It's normal to experience setbacks along the way, but with consistent effort and a willingness to learn from your experiences, you can enhance your ability to regulate your emotions, thoughts, and behaviors. You can learn how to listen to, confront, and manage your inner critic instead of letting it control you.

4. Tell Your Inner Critic to Move On

This may sound silly, but you can respond to your inner critic in the moment with a simple thought, such as *Okay, I hear you, but I don't want to listen to this, so I am going to move on*, or *No, but thank you for sharing*.

Treat your inner critic like you would a scared child. Acknowledge the small nudges it is sending you, but focus on your next steps to stop yourself from going into a downward spiral. The faster you acknowledge a thought, the easier it will be to move on from it, especially if you can use a healthy distraction in the moment to avoid ruminating, such as reading a book, working on a task, doing some yoga, going for a walk, listening to a podcast, or something similar.

Don't give in to the temptation to keep marinating in those thoughts. You can always come back to them when you feel calmer and less overwhelmed or stressed, using the table and questions above to work through your self-talk and get to the root of your thinking so you can start reframing how you see yourself.

5. Shift Your Focus

Get into the habit of reminding yourself that you are way more capable and valuable than your inner critic says you are. Remind yourself that it is possible to learn how to work with your inner critic and manage it while still recognizing your own importance and self-worth and trusting your decisions.

Below are some useful ways to practice this in the moment:

- When you have bad thoughts about yourself, try looking in the mirror and saying, "I want to believe that I am not [negative thought]."
- Practice saying this to yourself: "This [negative thought] is not who I am. I am just dealing with an unhealthy thought in my mind, and I am doing something about it. I am making it healthy."
- Picture yourself in your favorite place doing your favorite activity—do this whenever you feel the negative self-talk start to take hold again.

To download the table from this chapter, visit helpinahurrybook.com/resources

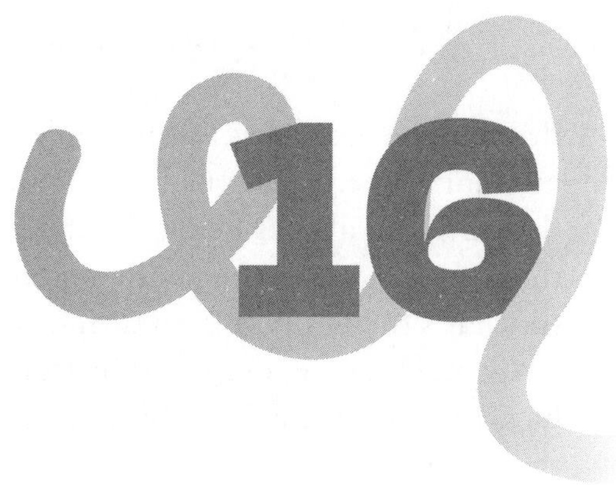

16

Help, I'm Self-Diagnosing Again!

Labels can be pretty amazing. They help us gain a sense of control over a situation, even if it's only the spice drawer in our kitchen. Applying a label can feel incredibly therapeutic—everything else may be falling apart around us, but at least this one part of our life is organized, systematized, and categorized.

When it comes to our mind, labeling what we are experiencing may feel equally therapeutic at first. When our mind feels like a hot mess, and our life looks equally tumultuous, putting a name and reason to our pain can feel like a godsend . . . until it isn't.

Mental health labels are a double-edged sword. They can give us something to hold on to, but they can also lock us in, taking the complexities of our life and stories and trying to put them in a neat box that cannot fully contain the depth and breadth of what we experience as human beings going through the messiness of life. They can quickly become dehumanizing, trapping us in our pain and making us think that this will always be our life because there is just something intrinsically wrong with our biology. We are "broken," so what's the point of even trying?

As much as we love classifications and systems, we also have to respect that they have their limits—and they have their sting, especially when they follow us into job applications or insurance eligibility or lead us into being too afraid to talk about how we feel because we fear we will be seen as "crazy." Labels may give a little comfort, but we have to be careful not to see them as an end point or use them to avoid managing our mind.

Yes, it is wonderful that we are so much more aware of mental health as a society and also much more open to talking about it in public and private spaces. On the other hand, alongside this awareness is a rise in people self-diagnosing and self-labeling their pain, especially online, which can end up causing a lot of distress for people who think, because they saw a TikTok video, that they have *x* and will have to live with it for the rest of their lives.[1]

Being constantly bombarded with certain types of mental health messaging can lead many people, especially children and teenagers, to interpret milder forms of distress as mental health problems by seeing themselves through the more reductionistic lens of a label, reducing the complexity of their experiences to "there must be something wrong with my biology" while disregarding the impact of their environment on the way they experience life. This, in turn, can cause individuals to experience a genuine increase in mental ill-health symptoms because how we think about ourselves and perceive our health can have real, physical impacts on our health due to the mind-brain-body connection.

As I have reiterated throughout this book, whatever we think about the most grows, and we merge with our environments. This means that labels are never just labels—by accepting a label, we merge with it as we think about it, which will affect how we perceive ourselves and our well-being. For example, increasingly seeing mild distress as symptomatic can reduce our tolerance and resilience, causing us to actually feel more distress in a wider range of situations than we would have previously and exacerbating our feelings of stress, anxiety, and overwhelm. If we are bombarded with the message that we have a low threshold for negative emotional experiences and a poor or a reduced ability to self-regulate our emotions, then this is what we will be more inclined to believe, reducing our ability to feel better mentally and physically.[2]

More and more researchers have been studying this phenomenon. Lucy Foulkes at the University of Oxford, for example, was one of the main psychologists involved in developing the idea of "prevalence inflation," which is used to explain, to a degree, how the increase in mental health messaging may lead to worse mental health outcomes.[3] Even though there have been extensive efforts in the West over the past several decades to raise public awareness around mental health problems, it appears that these issues have actually increased, not decreased as was first assumed.[4] Prevalence inflation tries to understand why this is the case, including why social media in particular tends to exacerbate this trend. Foulkes suggests, based on her research, that the bombardment of mental health messaging to raise awareness has in many ways made things worse because people tend to increasingly associate their negative emotions and experiences with mental illness as opposed to simply how we all experience life's ups and downs. This association can lead to increased self-diagnosis and self-labeling and decreased capacity to handle the normal turbulence of life.

More and more journalists are also reporting on this problem.[5] A recent article by Zoe Cunniffe titled "The TikTokification of Mental Health on Campus" is just one example. Cunniffe notes how

> Young adults on college campuses and elsewhere are being persuaded to interpret their everyday lives through the lens of mental illness as algorithms target them repeatedly with ads and other content. . . . [This] "marketing" encourages self-diagnosis and the embrace of disorders as identity by watering down the definition of mental suffering—and, paradoxically, minimizing understanding and compassion for those who are truly struggling.[6]

The statistics are staggering: TikTok posts tagged with #mentalhealth have over 100 billion views, and over 60 percent of people seeing these posts are under thirty years of age.[7] This prevalence of self-diagnosis can be incredibly problematic. It can encourage the oversharing of deep issues with people you don't know well online, and it tends to glamorize mental health challenges while making it harder for many people who are struggling to get the kind of help they need.[8]

There is also a lot of mental health misinformation out there, which further exacerbates these issues.[9] So many of us are online, which means that we are all susceptible to mental health misconceptions and misinformation.

Of course, it is not all bad news when it comes to mental health and social media. There is a sizable body of research showing evidence that social media engagement can be a source of community to rely on when connection is hard to find.[10] Social media use can provide a range of healthy social, developmental, and emotional benefits, such as making a way for connections with others, increasing understanding of oneself, and increasing a sense of connection between present and past selves.[11]

Candice Odgers, associate dean for research and a professor of psychological science and informatics at UC Irvine, is one of the key researchers in this area.[12] She notes how it is important to "*not* send the message to families—and to teens—that social-media use, which is common among adolescents and helpful in many cases, is inherently damaging, shameful, and harmful."[13] She notes how a lot of people can find "spaces of refuge online, especially when they have marginalized identities or lack support in their family and school."[14] Reality is a lot more complicated than we often think, especially when it comes to mental health awareness, labeling, and support.

At the end of the day, *how* we use social media and engage with and respond to mental health information are key. We each develop individual patterns of thinking and acting based on what we have gone through and what we are experiencing in the present, which impacts how we engage with our environment and how it impacts us, whether online or in real life.

This is especially the case when it comes to labels and self-diagnosis. If we are feeling locked in and trapped by what we see, hear, or read, we need to pause and ask ourselves why, and we must think about how we merge with our environments and how they can impact our ability to manage both everyday tasks and major life issues.

If you feel like this is an issue in your life, below are several strategies you can use to manage your feelings in the moment so that you can truly heal rather than trapping yourself in a label or diagnosis based on what someone else is telling you.

1. Check Your Headspace When You Engage

If you are in a negative mental space when you engage with mental health information, you will be more likely to make poor and reactive decisions that will have negative outcomes, especially if you are scrolling aimlessly online or through social media. You won't necessarily analyze what you are reading/watching and may end up ruminating on the negative, making it a reality in your life.

So, whenever you feel like a label or diagnosis describes "exactly" what you are going through, ask yourself:

- How am I mentally at this moment?
- Am I in a neutral mental space where I can handle what I am engaging with?

If you are not in a neutral mental space, take a break and shift your focus so you do not end up ruminating on what is "potentially" an issue, which can quickly become a self-fulfilling prophecy, crippling your natural resilience. Try to do something more constructive, like reading a book, working on a task you need to complete, going for a walk, texting a friend, or something else that helps you disengage from the negative.

2. Think About How You Think

In our technological age, it is easy to get caught up in shallow thinking. We are exposed to so much information at lightning speeds, often without the necessary tools or skills to process and understand what we are engaging with or exposing ourselves to.

The progression into an information era with easy access to endless streams of knowledge has changed how we think, feel, and make choices. In many cases, it's as if we have entered an era where we've sacrificed the need to process knowledge critically for the sake of gathering more and more data. We are, without realizing it, training ourselves not to think deeply but to jump to solutions and embrace opinions reactively as "facts."

However, gathering information without processing and applying it is counter to how our mind works and how the brain is structured. It can have a deleterious effect on our mental and physical well-being and health, which is why it is so important we practice deep thinking as much as possible. This can have many positive effects in our life, not just when it comes to self-diagnosing our pain and struggles.

To start practicing this in your life, the first step is to become more aware of how you think. Are you good at gathering data—scrolling from one headline, meme, post, comment, article, or piece of information to the next without stopping to think about what you are reading and looking at—and how is it impacting you? If so, how often are you doing this? How is it affecting your perception of yourself and your mental health? Writing down how often you do this can be an incredibly helpful way of tracking your behavior and what you need to work on.

As your awareness increases, practice deep thinking as much as you can to make it more of a habit. One of the best and easiest ways to do this is to choose something that interests you and really think about it in an intentional and deliberate way. *What is this saying? What does this mean? Why do I find this interesting? Is there a counterargument or different point of view, and, if so, which do I find more convincing?*

You can do this with any piece of information, such as a book chapter or article, a podcast, a documentary, and so on. The key is to really engage in a slow and deliberate way, without giving in to the temptation to come to an immediate, quick conclusion or skip something to get ahead.

3. Accept That Your Journey Will Look Different

We often set ourselves up for failure when we try to understand or follow someone else's healing journey. That's one reason the wellness industry can be so dangerous: Many people assert that healing and health come only when certain rules (created by them) are followed in a certain way.

But, as I have been saying throughout this book, we are all different and we all have different life experiences that have shaped who we are. Each of us has a veritable complex universe in our heads that simple explanations, labels, and solutions often fail to account for.

When it comes to what you need, how you heal, how you overcome challenges, and how you face what is holding you back both in the moment and long-term, remember that you set the playing field. You are writing your own story. Yes, you can learn from others, but if you constantly compare and contrast your life to what someone else is doing or saying, you can quickly lose sight of what makes you *you* and what you truly need to move forward.

4. Recognize That Labels Are Not Great Coping Mechanisms

Your experience doesn't need to be validated by a label or diagnosis. Your distress doesn't need to be defined as a disease. Your mental health struggles are not your entire identity, even if they make you feel like they are at times. When you are struggling, keep reminding yourself that even though things are tough, and even though life feels pretty dark and difficult right now, your negative feelings and thoughts are normal—they are *human*.

Your story is not an "it" to be diagnosed and labeled. What you are going through right now—these feelings are warning signals, telling you that something is going on that you need to address. The more you can acknowledge and embrace these warning signals, the faster you can get to the root of what you are experiencing and heal.

This doesn't mean that mental ill-health doesn't have real, physical effects on the brain and body. Of course these are impacted; the mind is moving through the brain and body and impacting your physiology and neurophysiology right down to your DNA. But you don't need a label or diagnosis to validate your pain, because what you are feeling is valid regardless of what someone else says.

So try not to use a label as a coping mechanism, as it can quickly lock you in rather than freeing you up to embrace what you are going through. If you have been labeled, or feel like you meet certain criteria, use this information to better understand where you are in life and what you need, and as a stepping stone to better understand how to seek help to manage your life for the better.

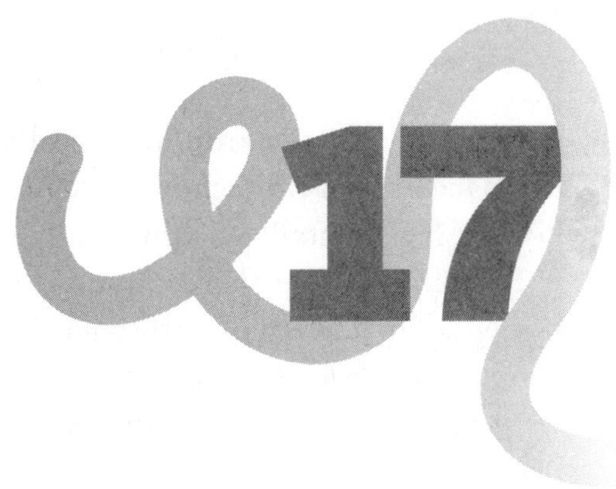

Help, Technology Is Everywhere!

I think we can all agree that technology is a double-edged sword. It can keep us connected but also disconnected. It can help us do our work but also distract us. It can bring us joy but also make us depressed. It can help us maintain our health but also adversely affect our well-being.

I don't think I need to list the thousands of articles, studies, and other sources of information that talk about the pros and cons of using technology in our world today. We are all in the thick of it, especially with the rise of artificial intelligence and how quickly it has become a part of our day-to-day lives. A year ago, I hardly heard anyone talk about ChatGPT except those in the know. Now? It's everywhere.

When it comes to technology use and how it affects us, an important thing to remember is that the brain is *plastic*, which means it is always changing. This means that we merge with both our external and internal environments—we adapt and absorb what is around us and what is within us. The fast pace of modern technology can have a major impact on how we feel mentally and physically—if we don't manage it.

However, we are also unique, which means that technology will impact each of us differently, whether we are talking about how we sleep, our mood, how we think, how distracted we get, and so on. I am a bit wary of applying too many blanket statements about the effects of technology on our health and well-being, as there is a lot of conflicting advice and research out there, and what may work for one person may not work for another.

Let's just look at the example of sleep and technology use. As technology advances, our sleep duration decreases. Or so we have been told. But are these two phenomena directly connected? And does this apply to all age groups? When it comes to our circadian rhythm, is screen time always a bad thing?

Many people have experienced a level of this happening in their lives. However, evidence gathered over the past ten years has actually shown that the link between technology and sleep is much more nuanced and complex than originally thought.[1] In fact, the mechanisms commonly thought to explain why technology use could cause sleep problems, mainly through arousal and bright light, are not well supported by research.[2] Most of the attention in researching this link between sleep and technology use has been given to adolescents and young adults, and studies in younger children and older adults are lacking, even though we know that different ages are affected by screen time and technology use in different ways.[3]

It seems that it's not so much the tech but rather how we are *managing* the tech. This is why it's important to figure out how to tailor or customize the recommendations on technology use and sleep to what we need and when. However, as reporter Alex Janin notes,

> This certainly doesn't give a free pass to spend hours glued to a phone before bed. Some people might be more sensitive to blue light than others. And certain people won't be bothered by engaging content, like video games, while others will find that even reading a printed book keeps them up.[4]

When it comes to technology use and sleep, a key thing we need to remember is that technology is designed to keep us engaged, entertained, and in a flow state where we lose track of time, and this will affect us in different ways.

This is why we have to look at our life in context: the big picture and the details. To once again use the example of sleep and technology use, and how "bad" screen time may be for our sleep patterns, we need to ask ourselves questions like, *Did I have sleep problems already that technology has made worse, or did using technology cause my sleep problems?*

Some researchers have even suggested that for some people, using technology before sleep might be helpful as a way to fill time and/or as an emotional regulation strategy to help them get to sleep.[5] For instance, the comfort of a favorite TV show just before sleep may do wonders for one person—and keep someone else up all night.[6]

I think the key thing we need to acknowledge is that technology is here to stay. When it comes to our health and well-being, we need to learn how to manage it rather than restrict it, and we can make it work for us. This means trying to avoid fear factors like "This is what your brain will look like after you watch *x* amount of TV or go on social media," understanding that research on technology use is still developing, and thinking about our own life and needs in context.

If you find that technology use is distracting you, stressing you out, and impacting your well-being, but you are not sure how to fix this, it is best to look at each situation you face individually, as just cutting all technology out of your life may not be a luxury you can afford or even want when all is said and done.

Below are several "help in a hurry" action steps you can take if you feel overwhelmed by technology and are not sure what to do at the moment. Not all of these tips may apply to you, and that is perfectly okay. You may find that some will help you find balance in your life at the moment, some may be useful in the future, and some may help someone you know. As I keep saying, we are all different and have different needs when it comes to how, when, and why we use technology, and how big of a role it plays in our life.

1. Notice Your Technology Habits

Observe yourself for several days, making note of how much you use technology. The average person spends up to eight hours a day using technology, while research indicates that some of the worst effects of electronic devices seem to be mitigated when devices are used less.[7]

If this sounds like you, and you are finding that you are battling being "online" so much, think of ways to limit or change your use of technology throughout the day. Some great ideas to consider are swapping out your e-reader for a paper book; listening to a podcast, music, or an audiobook instead of watching TV; going outdoors more during your free time; playing with your family or pets more; taking notes on paper instead of using your computer or smartphone; or mitigating some of the more intensive effects of screen time, such as by wearing specific light-blocking glasses.

2. Watch How You Sleep

If you feel like technology is affecting your sleeping pattern at night, take the time to work out your unique sleep pattern. Try keeping a log of your sleep habits for a week, including what technology you used and for how long, and how you felt the following day.

Below is a simple table you can use to track this, which you can also download using the QR code at the end of the chapter.

My Sleep Pattern

Day	How long did it take me to fall asleep?	What tech did I use, and for how long?	How did I feel the following day? How would I rate the quality of my rest?
Monday			
Tuesday			
Wednesday			
Thursday			
Friday			
Saturday			
Sunday			

If you feel that your technology use is specifically affecting the quality and quantity of your rest at night, think of ways you can reduce or change the way you use your time before bed and when you wake up. Some ways to do this include:

- Being very selective about what you watch at bedtime, if TV is an important part of your routine. Stick to calming, relaxing, humorous, and fictional content that is less engaging, and be careful of those cliffhangers and scary shows. Remember that all technology is designed to keep us engaged, entertained, and in a flow state where we lose track of time, so awareness of what you are watching and for how long is key.
- Many people find it helpful to leave technology out of the bedroom. If you choose to keep technology in the bedroom, put your devices in flight mode or do not disturb mode or turn off all unimportant notifications.
- Set a regular window of time for going to bed and rising, which helps regulate your circadian rhythm.
- Be aware of the algorithms targeting you to keep you engaged. This awareness will help you make better decisions regarding the amount of time you spend online and what you choose to engage with before bed.
- Try to avoid checking social media before bed or when you wake up. Worry and anxiety over missing out can result in negative arousal patterns before bed and can disrupt your ability to fall asleep, while starting your day off engaging with technology like social media or even emails first thing in the morning can upset you and affect your mood and ability to do what you need to do that day.

- Consider using an app or extension that helps you reduce how much time you spend on social media, like Forest, which helps you stay focused by planting virtual trees that grow while you stay away from your phone. If you leave the app to visit a social media site, your tree stops growing and can wither away. Another company I really like is StayFocusd, which is a browser extension that limits the amount of time you can spend on time-wasting websites. Think of ways you can incorporate these or something similar in your life.

3. Take More Thinker Moments

As mentioned in previous chapters, when we take time to switch off to what's going on around us and just think, we improve our ability to focus, our creativity, and our mood. Daydreaming or just letting our mind wander is something we should all be doing on a regular basis, and it can help us mitigate some of the more negative effects technology can have on us if we feel overwhelmed, stressed out, forgetful, or distracted.

It is also something we can do quickly in the moment, and it helps calm down the mind-brain-body network. This can be really helpful for those situations where we have to engage with technology, like at work or school, or when we feel particularly stressed out by being online, say if we are triggered on social media or by watching TV.

Here's how you can have a thinker moment just a few times each day (or as often as you need):

1. Think of yourself as the actor, director, screenwriter, and audience of a mental performance—*your* mental

performance. Now, simply close your eyes and let your mind wander.

2. You can start the process by intentionally thinking of something pleasant and meaningful, and then let this lead you into a flow of thoughts. Prompt yourself with topics you'd find rewarding to daydream about, like a pleasant memory, a future accomplishment, or an event you're looking forward to.
3. Be observant about what you are thinking about. Indeed, as you take a "thinker moment," you may be surprised to notice what thoughts and feelings pop up from your nonconscious during these moments. Don't panic; this is perfectly normal. Just take note of them and plan to address them later—try to avoid ruminating on them and letting them interrupt your internal rest time.
4. As you daydream, you can listen to some music, take a walk outside, or doodle. These moments can last any length of time from a short ten seconds to a full hour. Trust that it's possible to have a good experience if you prime your brain with topics you find pleasant.

Thinker moments are something all of us can do once we have the concept, even children. Daydreaming makes sense to us, no matter our age.

When I want to have a thinker moment, I personally like to just stop and stare out a window for a few seconds. I find this very helpful and invigorating—especially when I am really stressed or anxious or am in the middle of a busy workday. If possible, I also try to go outside; being in nature and getting that vitamin D really takes that thinker moment to the next level!

4. Build Your Brain

Instead of spending hours on social media or just scrolling aimlessly online, take the time to think deeply and build your brain. You don't necessarily have to "quit" technology to do this. Just schedule in some time to read a section in a book (fiction or nonfiction), read an article or a study, or listen to a podcast or part of an audiobook and think deeply about the information you have just received. Ask yourself what the author or authors are trying to say, answer your question by writing down several points, and discuss what you have learned with a family member, friend, or colleague.

Thinking deeply about information fires up our mind, helping us become more resilient, feel less overwhelmed, think more clearly, and build healthy memories. This is a great way to counteract the more negative, mind-spiraling effects of technology use that many of us experience, and it is something we can all do quite easily—no need to invest thousands of dollars in the latest device or object designed to protect us from the negative effects of the modern online age.

To download the table from this chapter, visit helpinahurrybook.com/resources

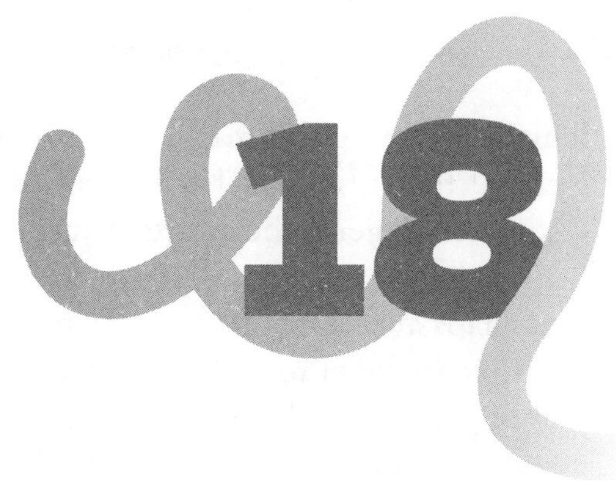

18

Help, Everything Is Going Wrong!

When I started writing this book, there was one thing that consistently came up when I spoke to people about what they felt like they needed help with on a day-to-day basis, and that was the unexpected chaos of life. When things just go wrong, what do you do? When you are hit with bad news, how do you handle it? When everything bad, everything you dread, happens all at once, how do you escape the storm?

We have all experienced these moments in life, times when clichéd phrases like "The night is darkest before the dawn" and "There's a light at the end of the tunnel" seem ridiculous and even taunting. How could things ever be better? Perhaps you are experiencing this right now and have grabbed this book as a last resort. How do you get out of this tunnel? How do you make it to the dawn?

It doesn't help that there is so much going on in the world around us, all the time—it is easy to feel overwhelmed and like everything is a mess. Yes, it is so much easier to stay connected these days, but this is a mixed blessing. It is also so much easier to be aware of just how terrible this world and humanity can truly be, which can compound our sense of chaos and desperation in the moment.

Like we want to regain a sense of control when we face uncertainty, we also want to do so when confronted with bad news, but control often feels elusive and unattainable. I think we all know, deep down, that there is so much we cannot control, and when things are going badly, we are forced to confront this reality without the "padding" of stability or happiness.

However, as I have mentioned throughout this book, the one thing we can control is how we choose to respond to what curveballs life throws at us. This is not easy or simple to do, but it is worth the effort, as it does more than just give us back some level of control over what is happening; it can give us a sense of peace amid the chaos of life, which is invaluable.

Maintaining a sense of peace when the world feels like it is falling apart around us is truly one of the most incredible skills we can develop as human beings because so much in life is unexpected, uncertain, and painful. Peace is like fuel. It helps us get through the darkness. It helps us *see*, not with our eyes but *with our mind*. It brings a sense of clarity and wisdom to a situation. Without fuel or energy from a battery, a car can't move—it's stuck. Without a sense of peace, we get stuck. But if we can hang on to a sense of peace while everything is a mess? This is priceless.

Peace in the midst of chaos doesn't mean that we are happy when bad things happen to us, or that we just accept the discomfort, pain, and heartache without fighting back. It also doesn't mean we turn a blind eye to what we are experiencing or try to suppress our more uncomfortable or distressing emotions.

Part of practicing peace is recognizing that it is okay to struggle—that it is okay not to be okay, which is a key theme in this book. It means learning how to be at peace with who we are, where we are, and where we want to be, even if right now things seem so terrible. One of my favorite authors and artists, Morgan Harper Nichols, describes this brilliantly: "Peace is a state of mind, heart, body, and soul. It is the freedom to breathe, even in the face of great challenges and chaos. Peace is the river in the desert, not on the other side of it."[1]

We experience this kind of peace on a nonconscious level before we feel "at peace" physically. In the brain, it shows as nonconscious activity in the deepest, most intelligent, and insightful parts of us *before* it's even experienced consciously. It increases coherence between the hemispheres of the brain, helping us function better both mentally and physically so we can respond to and overcome the challenges of life. It is, in a way, the kind of peace poets or philosophers would describe as "soul deep"—the ultimate form of control.

If we seek out peace when we are first faced with bad news, we are tuning in to the depths of who we are and changing our brain and body's responses accordingly. This helps us develop a mindset that says, "I will be okay. Somehow, I will get through this." This is not something we just tell ourselves to feel better; it is something we *know*, something that truly makes us feel more in control regardless of what we are facing. In fact, just thinking about experiencing peace—drawing on that deepness of the soul even when we receive bad news or when life feels chaotic—can shift our perception and even alter our brain and body's chemistry and structure in a positive direction so we can somehow cope.[2]

I would even say that if you skip every other chapter in this book and only read this one, then you will already be more prepared to handle the ups and downs of life than you were before, which is really what this book is all about and is a fitting epilogue to the power of harnessing your incredible mind, brain, and body to deal with challenges in the moment.

So, how do you do this? How do you find that elusive "river in the desert," especially when everything suddenly, unavoidably, and completely falls apart? It all starts—and ends—with how you manage your mind (your thoughts, feelings, and choices) in the moment, which will take practice and time, so don't feel disheartened if you fall prey to the chaos when you first start trying to seek out peace. This is part of the journey, and it just emphasizes the fact that you are, like the rest of us, only human. Remind yourself that it is okay not to be okay, that it is okay to struggle, and that even when you feel down and trampled by life, this sense of peace is still within your grasp; it's in the depths of your soul.

Below are several tips to help you practice finding this sense of peace and control when faced with the bad or the unexpected. These strategies can be applied to all the chapters above, too, as well as any other issue you have to face in the moment that steers you away from the safe harbor of peace.

1. Practice Deep Breathing to Center Yourself

When we are faced with something bad or unexpected, it can be hard to even think straight, let alone practice a visualization or grounding exercise or utilize a strategy to find peace in the midst of the chaos of life. This is where following our instinct to breathe deeply is worth channeling in an organized way because that soul-deep peace truly is a breath away. Deep breathing calms down your mind, brain, and body and should be done before you try any of the following strategies.

This is such a simple thing to practice that it may seem silly in the face of the unexpected, but how you breathe is so incredibly powerful, as I've mentioned throughout this book. It is always worth reminding ourselves that just changing the way we inhale and exhale can transform a single moment into an opportunity to find peace even when we feel trapped or overwhelmed.

As you inhale and exhale, your heart rate increases and decreases, respectively. This is called heart rate variability (HRV), and a higher HRV is beneficial, as it can increase the resilience of your stress-response system.[3] In states of high anxiety and toxic stress, like when the unexpected or bad happens, our HRV generally decreases, affecting our autonomic nervous system and how we handle stress.

Deep breathing is so helpful because it increases your HRV in the moment, allowing you to manage how you feel and gain that sense of "peace" more quickly and effectively. You can practice this by pacing your respiration to approximately five or six breaths per minute, which will help calm down your neurophysiology so that you can better manage what you are faced with.[4] I also find breathing in deeply for three counts and out for three counts helpful in these situations, or breathing in deeply for three counts and out slowly and forcefully for seven counts, if you find it hard to figure out how to breathe five to six times a minute.

EEG studies show that breathing exercises like these increase alpha frequency and decrease theta frequency power, which together will help you focus and think more clearly, even when surrounded by chaos.[5] The extra oxygen also helps to increase activity in the front and side of the brain and some structures like the hypothalamus and thalamus and part of the brain stem. Collectively, this helps with comfort, relaxation, pleasantness, vigor, and alertness as well as reduces symptoms of arousal, anxiety, depression, anger, and confusion—just what you need in times of trouble.

2. Visualize Your Tunnel

When you are in the middle of life's chaos, visualize a tunnel, the length and darkness of which you can determine based on what you are facing. What does this look like in your life? How does it represent what you are going through?

Next, visualize a light at the end of this tunnel. Clichéd, perhaps, but this imagery is so effective because it is something we can all grasp on some level. Try to imagine this in as much detail as possible, even if it is only a faint vision. You may even have an image of how you would like things to pan out, which is great. As your peace increases over time, so will the clarity of what you imagine.

You can take this exercise to a deeper level by imagining that the tunnel is filled with quicksand and you must navigate your way through it to get to the other side. Just think of what happens when people fall into quicksand. They get caught and begin sinking. They try to struggle out of the quicksand with rapid and stressful movements, which only makes them sink even more. The only way they manage to escape is through reaching for a vine to pull themselves out or a friend/companion throwing in a rope or something that they can use to pull themselves out. What will get you out of this quicksand tunnel? What will help you? Try to imagine this in as much detail as possible.

The purpose of this exercise is to find a simple way to visualize what you are facing and a way out of it—to regain some degree of control over the problem by "boxing it in" in this way and seeing a way out in your mind's eye as a positive expectation for your future. This, as mentioned above, actually charges up your mind, brain, and body for positive action, making you more prepared mentally and physically to face what you are dealing with in the moment.

Here, it is important to remind yourself that *peace does not equal happiness*. It does not always mean the chaos around you will end and you will be happy. It might just mean that you are able to keep your head above the "quicksand" of life and find time to breathe. Remember that, even if you are not there yet, there will be a time when things are better. Just like the good times do not last, the bad times come to an end too.

3. Reach Out

The reason I like the quicksand metaphor is because it serves as a perfect example of what it feels like to be overwhelmed by the chaos around you and within you—when you feel like you are sinking under the pressure of it all. And, just like someone struggling in quicksand must reach for something or someone to help them, you can learn how to navigate the "quicksand" of life and find peace by doing the same: reaching out.

This starts with acknowledging the level of stress that you are under; in other words, name what is stealing your peace. You can use this information to assess how you should move forward. What is your quicksand?

Next, you need to assess how fast you are sinking, how much of your body is going under, and what is around you that you can use to escape. Apply this in your life by asking yourself what you are feeling, saying, or doing when you feel overwhelmed and stuck. What is burying you? Can you ask for help? Can you speak to someone? Can you change something? What can you do to reach out?

I understand that this last part is often easier said than done. Asking for help can be one of the hardest things for us to do, especially when we are struggling emotionally. It can also be hard to recognize when we need help and can't just "get through it." It can feel sad, frustrating, or even weak to think that sometimes we just aren't "strong" enough. In a society that often prioritizes independence and power, asking for help often seems like a silly or even bad thing. This doesn't mean you must trust just anyone; tune in to yourself and trust yourself, and you will know who to reach out to and when.

The important thing to remember is not to beat yourself up if you get to this point. We have all been there and will most likely get there again along life's path. Practice self-compassion, grace, and kindness, and try to see asking for help as something that's both incredibly hard and incredibly powerful. It is not a sign of weakness or failure.

Someone once told me about a type of experiential therapy that changed their whole perspective about asking for help.[6] They were part of a group of people from all areas and backgrounds. Some were alcoholics and others drug addicts; some had suffered sexual trauma and others had severe mental health problems. These people had gotten to a place in their lives where they were so broken by what they were going through that it became hard to even participate in normal life. They were going to group therapy to try to learn how to cope with everything.

One day in therapy, they did this activity: The therapists blindfolded everyone and told them they were going to enter a maze made from ropes. The therapists also explained that everyone had to hold on to the ropes—they must not let go. The "rope maze" was set up prior to the beginning of the activity, so the participants did not know what to expect. Once their hands were on the rope, they were given a set of instructions, including that they must keep at least one hand on the rope and must be silent.

During this session, the participants would slowly start looking for a way out. They followed the person in front of them—and went in circles. Around and around and around again. Some people would think they found their way out only to realize they were still in the circle. Every five minutes, the therapist repeated, "Remember, there is a way out . . . raise your hand if you think you've found the exit or if you need help." During the last five minutes of the activity, the therapist played the Beatles' song "Help!" as a clue to help them exit the maze.

The point of this activity was that there was no true end to the maze if the participants kept trying to leave on their own. The only way out of the maze was to raise a hand and ask for help. Yet the participants were so focused on the rules that they completely disregarded the final bit where the therapist said, "Raise your hand if you need help." If they raised their hand and asked for help, the therapist took their hand off the rope and helped them remove their blindfold so they could see that they had just been following the same pattern in the rope maze—they had just been going in circles.

I think this is something everyone can relate to. We tend to think that asking for help is a sign of weakness and being self-reliant is what makes us successful. But this is simply not true. When we acknowledge that we can't do something alone, it is a sign of both humility and strength. We are strong enough to admit that we don't have all the answers. This doesn't make us weak. It makes us human!

So, if you are struggling, remind yourself that you need to be connected not only to survive but also to thrive. Remind yourself of this rope maze activity. You don't have to feel guilty if you need to reach out to others. This brings perspective and will help you move through and overcome the issues of life. These kinds of connections will positively impact your health, right down to the level of your genetic expression.

4. Take Action

To build on the quicksand imagery above, think about what "vines" you can grab on to in order to keep from sinking into the chaos you are experiencing. Write down your answers to help organize your thinking, trying to be as specific as possible. How exactly can you implement these changes in your life?

Here are some examples:

- Establish clear boundaries to protect your time, energy, and emotional well-being. Learn to say no. Learn to delegate *and* practice not feeling guilty when doing so.
- Tell yourself often that it's okay not to be okay. Put reminders of this where you will see them throughout your day.
- Prioritize your mental self-care. How can you strengthen your mental health and resilience when times are good so you have a "vine" to pull on when you find yourself falling into the quicksand of life? For instance, you can participate in relaxation

techniques like taking a bath, practicing yoga, or enjoying hobbies that help you unwind and find time to rest and restore.

- Maintain a consistent daily routine that includes exercise, proper nutrition, and adequate sleep. Physical health is closely tied to mental and emotional well-being.
- Take regular breaks from digital devices and social media to disconnect from external chaos and reconnect with yourself. Getting out in nature is one of my favorite ways to do this.
- Talk to a trusted friend, family member, or therapist about your feelings and experiences. Sharing your thoughts and concerns with someone you trust can provide comfort and perspective.
- While limiting exposure to negative information is essential, it's also important to stay informed about important events. Find a balanced approach that allows you to stay informed without being overwhelmed.

5. Don't Marinate in Your Feelings

This is key: Constantly focusing on how you feel without managing it can seriously impact your ability to find peace in the chaos. Yes, it is important to acknowledge, not suppress, how you feel, but you need to do this in a balanced way or you can exacerbate your feelings of being trapped, which will really steal your peace. Ruminating on the negative is kind of like panicking if you find yourself trapped in quicksand: You will only sink further.

This is why it is important to review what you're experiencing as logically as possible, and a great way to do this is using what I call the "camera exercise" to ground you in the moment and help you focus:

1. Find a place to sit comfortably and then close your eyes. Take a few deep breaths to help calm down your mind, brain, and body.
2. Now, visualize the past few hours, days, or weeks, as if you were scrolling through your camera looking at photos and videos, for one to two minutes. You are focusing on how you felt prior to the issue you are facing now, almost as if what you are going through hasn't happened yet. This is the "review" stage of the exercise.
3. Next, focus on the present moment—what you are doing, feeling, and experiencing right now—for one to two minutes. What has happened to steal your peace? This is the "occupy" stage, where you are occupying the moment and trying to figure out what happened and how you feel in as logical a way as possible.
4. Lastly, think about how you want to feel about what happened or how you want this to play out in your future or even the next hour (whatever time frame you choose for the situation). This is the "observe" step, where you are shifting your focus from how you feel to what you are going to do about what has happened. How will you regain your sense of peace in the chaos? Do this for one to two minutes.

6. Think About the Good Times and Practice Gratitude

As I mentioned in chapter 2, our memories are more than just memories; they are a physical part of us and can help strengthen our psychoneurobiology and our ability to handle the chaos of life. How?

When we choose to focus on the good we have experienced, we increase the positive emotions inside our memory networks, which are the "glue" keeping our memories together inside the thought. This, in turn, "turbo-boosts" the happy memory, shooting it to the conscious mind so that it demands attention, but in a good way.

This process can increase our sense of hope, peace, and resilience in the moment, which, in turn, can help bring clarity, perspective, and wisdom when we are experiencing a challenge. It also helps reduce toxic, unmanaged stress, while the activity of recalling the happy thoughts reactivates the imagination and boosts our psychoneurobiology, which is the way our mind, brain, and body connect and work together.

This includes being grateful for what we have experienced in life. Research on the effects gratitude has on our biology shows how being thankful increases our longevity, our ability to use our imagination, and our ability to problem-solve.[7] Gratitude is deeply powerful because it makes us feel that life is worth living even when we are faced with the bad or unexpected.[8]

So, if you are facing something particularly hard, have just been told some very bad news, or feel like everything is falling apart around you, take the time to acknowledge how you feel while also choosing to remind yourself of the happy times in your life and what you have to be grateful for. This is not replacing the negative with the positive or trying to get rid of any bad feelings you are experiencing; rather, it is using happy memories and the joy you have experienced in life, or what you have to be thankful for, to strengthen your mind and brain in the moment so that you can better focus on and deal with what is causing you distress. It is using the "good" to increase your resilience to the "bad," almost like building a bridge, which can help you be okay with not being okay, as I have mentioned in previous chapters.

I would liken this to an insurance policy. In the same way you take out insurance on your home and life to prepare for the unexpected, you can take out "insurance" for the way you react to life. Just think for a moment about what insurance is: protection against a possible eventuality. You can deliberately and intentionally live in a way that recognizes the unexpected and painful will happen, and you will get thrown and upset, but because you have built insurance policy networks into your psychoneurobiology, you have opened the door to your unlimited resilience and so will draw on these in the time of crisis.

In this way, in all the challenges of life, you can apply the words of Maya Angelou, the renowned American author and poet: "I can be changed by what happens to me. But I refuse to be reduced by it."[9] More specifically, at the brain level, building insurance policy networks does the following:

1. It prompts a healthy, balanced brain wave flow, with bursts of healing theta energy waves.
2. It activates the amygdala, which is like a library keeping your emotional perceptions in "books." This helps you develop healthy emotional perceptions that enhance the overall functionality of the amygdala.
3. It activates the frontal cortex, which can improve blood flow and coherence between the two sides of the brain. This can improve your resilience, decision-making abilities, and intelligence.
4. It switches on the different components of the mirror neuron system in the inferior frontal/premotor

and inferior parietal cortex as you experience the increased bonding and sharing that come from talking about a happy memory with your loved ones.

5. It increases your sense of imagination, which means new thoughts with new memories are being built into the brain, strengthening it while also increasing your resilience. It is almost as though good memories build a supportive lattice/network in the brain, which helps you stay strong during hard times (the ultimate insurance policy)!
6. It activates systems for reward and positive affect in the brain and body, including the ventral tegmental area, nucleus accumbens, and the orbitofrontal cortex.
7. It boosts serotonin and dopamine, which are neurotransmitters in the brain that give you feelings of satisfaction and well-being and cause the pleasure/reward centers in the brain to light up. Endorphins, which are the body's natural painkiller, also can be released when you think of happy times in the past or what you are grateful for.

Some great ways to build up your mind insurance policies by thinking about the good times and practicing gratitude are:

1. *Volunteer.* Find a local organization and join their volunteer team. When you help those in need, you will realize just how blessed you are.
2. *Meditate.* Start every morning meditating on what you are thankful for and memories that make you happy. Counting your blessings early in the day makes it easier to recognize them later because your

mind will get better and better at the process of building a positive and grateful mindset. Remember, the more good you see in your life in the "now moments," the happier and more successful you are likely to be at school, work, and life in the future.

3. *Pause.* Every time you find yourself feeling down or overwhelmed, think about all the good things in your life. Maybe write down what you are grateful for and what makes you happy on a sticky note and place it somewhere near you, or set up a reminder on your phone. Perhaps text or call a friend to tell them how thankful you are to have them in your life or just to share a happy memory and laugh together.
4. *Remember.* Below are some helpful mantras you can use to remind yourself that you will get through a dark or challenging time:
   - I don't know how I am going to get through this, but I have made it through tough times before. I will persevere.
   - I am not alone. I am not weak.
   - These moments will pass.
   - What's happened is behind me; what matters now is what I do going forward.
   - It's not worth sweating the small stuff.
   - I can get frustrated or upset, but if I don't limit the amount of time I allow myself to do so, I am just making it harder to move forward.

Conclusion

It's Okay Not to Be Okay

Phew! You made it through this book, and, if I can hazard a guess, more than a few tough situations in life. You may still feel like a mess or at least like life is still messy. *Same!*

What? Me? The mental health professional and clinical neuroscientist also has a messy life and mind at times? Yes! That's the thing about life: It is messy. And that's the thing about our mind: It's really good at managing messes, with practice and know-how.

I think too often we go through life thinking that it's not "good" to struggle, to feel pain, to be uncomfortable, or to feel like a #hotmess, as the saying goes. But the reality is we all feel this at times, even those of us who seem to have it all together on the surface.

The principles in this book? I use them every day. Indeed, half the time I was writing this book I felt like I was talking to myself! And saying those same phrases:

"I've had it up to here!"

"I can't take it anymore."

"My head's about to explode."
"Give me strength!"
"I give up!"
"Why me?"
"I am at the end of my rope."
"I am going to tear my hair out!"
"I am at a breaking point."
"I am sick with worry."
"I am an anxious wreck."
"This was the straw that broke the camel's back."
"I am climbing the walls!"
"It's all downhill from here."

But the other half the time? I have been reminding myself that though life is really tough, I am only human, and that it really is okay not to feel okay. Even if I don't have things all together right now, I am still writing my story. We all are! It's a journey in the making, and there will be ups for all those downs we are experiencing right now.

I have started really thinking about those sayings above and what they mean to me. And the more I work on managing my own stresses in the moment, the more I have found new, different phrases that speak to where I am and where I want to be at the moment:

"Some days you have to create your own sunshine."[1]
"A bad day is not a bad life."[2]
"Slow progress is better than no progress."[3]
"Oh yes, the past can hurt. But the way I see it, you can either run from it or learn from it."[4]

"In your life, where are you not making mistakes? Sometimes if there's no mess, there's no change happening."[5]

"Embrace each challenge in your life as an opportunity for self-transformation."[6]

"On the other side of a storm is the strength that comes from having navigated through it. Raise your sail and begin."[7]

"Turn your wounds into wisdom."[8]

The greatest advice I can give you on this wild, beautiful, and often painful adventure we call life is to treat yourself with kindness and self-compassion, especially in those moments when your life feels like it is falling apart. Be patient and *very* kind to yourself during challenging times. Try not to be too hard on yourself for feeling stressed or overwhelmed.

Remind yourself that things like chaos, sadness, pain, anger, and self-doubt are a part of life—but they do not have to take you out. They can, in fact, help you grow. The only person who decides when your story is over is *you*. So don't ever stop writing. The first few drafts (maybe many drafts!) are always a mess. But the end result? That is truly priceless. Don't let anyone, yourself included, tell you otherwise.

Notes

Chapter 1 Help in a Hurry, What's That?

1. Caroline Leaf et al., "Habit Formation and Automaticity: Psychoneurobiological Correlates of Gamma Activity," *NeuroRegulation* 11, no. 1 (2024): 2–24, https://www.neuroregulation.org/article/view/23416/14768.

2. Caroline Leaf, "Meet Dr. Caroline Leaf," accessed September 18, 2024, https://drleaf.com.

Chapter 2 Help, What's Going On in My Head?

1. Leaf et al., "Habit Formation and Automaticity"; Elissa S. Epel, "Telomeres in a Life-Span Perspective: A New 'Psychobiomarker'?" *Current Directions in Psychological Science* 18, no. 1 (2009): 6–10, https://doi.org/10.1111/j.1467-8721.2009.01596.x.

Chapter 3 Help, I'm Under Pressure!

1. Tim Chin, "How Pressure Cookers Actually Work," Serious Eats, May 7, 2023, https://www.seriouseats.com/how-pressure-cookers-work.

2. The original quote reads, "Results! Why, man, I have gotten a lot of results! I know several thousand things that won't work." Frank Lewis Dyer and Thomas Commerford Martin, *Edison: His Life and Inventions*, vol. 2 (Harper and Brothers, 1910), 616.

Chapter 4 Help, My Brain Won't Shut Up!

1. Rapid Transformational Therapy, "How to Stop Overthinking," *RTT Blog* (blog), September 24, 2024, https://rtt.com/how-to-stop-overthinking/; Susan Nolen-Hoeksema, "Most Women Think Too Much, Overthinkers Often Drink Too Much," University of Michigan News,

September 24, 2024, https://news.umich.edu/most-women-think-too-much-overthinkers-often-drink-too-much/.

2. Yasmin Anwar, "Social Scientists Build Case for 'Survival of the Kindest'," ScienceDaily, December 9, 2009, https://www.sciencedaily.com/releases/2009/12/091208155309.htm.

Chapter 5 Help, I Want to Punch That Person in the Face!

1. Kendall Magill, "19 Anonymous Quotes You NEED to Read," Odyssey, November 8, 2016, https://www.theodysseyonline.com/19-anonymous-quotes-you-need-to-read.

2. Ohio State University, "Breathe, Don't Vent: Turning Down the Heat Is Key to Managing Anger," ScienceDaily, March 18, 2024, www.sciencedaily.com/releases/2024/03/240318142352.htm.

Chapter 6 Help, the World Seems So Black-and-White!

1. Katharina Star, "How to Overcome All-or-Nothing Thinking," Verywell Mind, November 20, 2023, https://www.verywellmind.com/all-or-nothing-thinking-2584173.

2. Star, "How to Overcome All-or-Nothing Thinking."

Chapter 7 Help, I'm Tired All the Time!

1. Stuart Hameroff and Roger Penrose, "Consciousness in the Universe: An Updated Review of the 'Orch OR' Theory," *Physics of Life Reviews* 11, no. 1 (2014): 39–78, https://doi.org/10.1016/j.plrev.2013.08.002.

2. *Merriam-Webster*, "Restoring," accessed December 12, 2024, https://www.merriam-webster.com/dictionary/Restoring; *Merriam-Webster*, "Rest," accessed December 12, 2024, https://www.merriam-webster.com/dictionary/rest#dictionary-entry-2.

3. Daniel Klein, "'Law & Order' Actor Sam Waterston: What Quitting My Job After Nearly 20 Years Taught Me About Happiness," CNBC, June 13, 2024, https://www.cnbc.com/2024/06/13/sam-waterston-of-law-order-what-quitting-taught-me-about-happiness.html.

4. Klein, "'Law & Order' Actor Sam Waterston."

Chapter 8 Help, My Intrusive Thoughts Just Won't Quit!

1. Richard Moulding et al., "They Scare Because We Care: The Relationship Between Obsessive Intrusive Thoughts and Appraisals and Control Strategies Across 15 Cities," *Journal of Obsessive-Compulsive and Related Disorders* 3, no. 3 (March 2014): 280–91.

2. Caroline Leaf, *Cleaning Up Your Mental Mess: 5 Simple, Scientifically Proven Steps to Reduce Anxiety, Stress, and Toxic Thinking* (Baker Books, 2021).

3. Matthew L. Dixon et al., “Interactions Between the Default Network and Dorsal Attention Network Vary Across Default Subsystems, Time, and Cognitive States,” *NeuroImage* 147 (2017): 632–49.

Chapter 9 Help, I Don’t Feel Happy All the Time!

1. Vasundhara Sawhney, “It’s Okay to Not Be Okay,” *Harvard Business Review*, November 10, 2020, https://hbr.org/2020/11/its-okay-to-not-be-okay.

2. Sawhney, “It’s Okay to Not Be Okay”; Arizona State University, “It’s Okay When You’re Not Okay: A Re-evaluation of Resilience in Adults,” ScienceDaily, August 16, 2018, www.sciencedaily.com/releases/2018/08/180816091436.htm.

3. Joseph Henrich, “Q&A on WEIRD,” Harvard University, accessed September 18, 2024, https://weirdpeople.fas.harvard.edu/qa-weird.

4. Abigail Shrier, “Stop Constantly Asking Your Kids How They Feel,” *Wall Street Journal*, March 8, 2024, https://www.wsj.com/health/wellness/stop-constantly-asking-your-kids-how-they-feel-d36cf32e; Brett Q. Ford et al., “Culture Shapes Whether the Pursuit of Happiness Predicts Higher or Lower Well-Being,” *Journal of Experimental Psychology: General* 144, no. 6 (2015): 1053–62, https://doi.org/10.1037/xge0000108.

5. As quoted in Ford et al., “Culture Shapes.”

6. Ford et al., “Culture Shapes.”

7. Shigeyuki Takai et al., “Do People Who Highly Value Happiness Tend to Ruminate?” *Current Psychology* 42, (2023): 32443–55, https://doi.org/10.1007/s12144-022-04131-6.

8. Ford et al., “Culture Shapes.”

9. Harvard Second Generation Study, “Welcome to the Harvard Study of Adult Development,” Harvard Second Generation Study, accessed September 18, 2024, https://www.adultdevelopmentstudy.org.

10. Amy L. Gentzler et al., “Valuing Happiness in Youth: Associations with Depressive Symptoms and Well-Being,” *Journal of Applied Developmental Psychology* 66 (2019): 1–10, https://doi.org/10.1016/j.appdev.2019.03.001.

11. Springer, “Can Pursuing Happiness Make You Unhappy?,” Science Daily, March 12, 2018, www.sciencedaily.com/releases/2018/03/180312104036.htm.

12. Ashton Jackson, “The Happiest People Use These 3 Phrases Often, from Psychologists and Workplace Experts,” CNBC, June 23, 2024, https://www.cnbc.com/2024/06/23/phrases-happy-people-in-finland-denmark-often-use.html; The International, “Pyt Med Det! A Danish Way of Not Sweating the Small Stuff,” *The International*, June 2024, https://www.the-intl.com/post/pyt-med-det-a-danish-way-of-not-sweating-the-small-stuff.

13. Penn State, "Short-Term Loneliness Associated with Physical Health Problems," ScienceDaily, June 13, 2024, www.sciencedaily.com/releases/2024/06/240613140903.htm.

14. Jessica Martino, Jennifer Pegg, and Elizabeth Pegg Frates, "The Connection Prescription: Using the Power of Social Interactions and the Deep Desire for Connectedness to Empower Health and Wellness," *American Journal of Lifestyle Medicine* 11, no. 6 (2015): 466–75, https://pmc.ncbi.nlm.nih.gov/articles/PMC6125010/; Carrianne J. Leschak and Naomi I. Eisenberger, "Two Distinct Immune Pathways Linking Social Relationships with Health: Inflammatory and Antiviral Processes," *Psychosomatic Medicine* 81, no. 8 (2019): 711–19, https://pubmed31600173; Emma Seppala, "Connectedness & Health: The Science of Social Connection," Stanford University Center for Compassion and Altruism Research and Education, May 8, 2014, https://ccare.stanford.edu/uncategorized/connectedness-health-the-science-of-social-connection-infographic/.

Chapter 10 Help, I'm Angry All the Time!

1. Better Health Channel, "Anger: How It Affects People," Better Health Channel, accessed September 18, 2024, https://www.betterhealth.vic.gov.au/health/healthyliving/anger-how-it-affects-people.

2. Leaf et al., "Habit Formation and Automaticity."

3. Sarah N. Garfinkel et al., "Anger in Brain and Body: The Neural and Physiological Perturbation of Decision-Making by Emotion," *Social Cognitive and Affective Neuroscience* 11, no. 1 (2015): 150–58, https://www.ncbi.nlm.nih.gov/pmc/articles/PMC4692323/.

4. Garfinkel et al., "Anger in Brain and Body."

5. R. J. R. Blair, "Considering Anger from a Cognitive Neuroscience Perspective," *WIREs Cognitive Science* 3, no. 1 (2011): 65–74, https://www.ncbi.nlm.nih.gov/pmc/articles/PMC3260787/.

6. Paloma Moisii et al., "The Relationship Between Job Strain and Ischemic Heart Disease Mediated by Endothelial Dysfunction Markers and Imaging," *Medicina* 60, no. 7, (2024): 1048, https://doi.org/10.3390/medicina60071048.

7. Johns Hopkins Medicine, "For Your Heart: Stay Calm and Cool," Johns Hopkins Medicine, accessed September 18, 2024, https://www.hopkinsmedicine.org/health/wellness-and-prevention/for-your-heart-stay-calm-and-cool.

8. Stephen E. Lupe, Laurie Keefer, and Eva Szigethy, "Gaining Resilience and Reducing Stress in the Age of COVID-19," *Current Opinion in Gastroenterology* 36, no. 4 (2020): 295–303, https://pubmed.ncbi.nlm.nih.gov/32398567/.

Chapter 11 Help, My Regrets Are Holding Me Back!

1. Natasha Parikh, Felipe de Brigard, and Kevin S. LaBar, "The Efficacy of Downward Counterfactual Thinking for Regulating Emotional Memories in Anxious Individuals," *Frontiers in Psychology* 12 (2022): 712066, https://doi.org/10.3389/fpsyg.2021.712066.

2. Isabelle Bauer and Carsten Wrosch, "Making Up for Lost Opportunities: The Protective Role of Downward Social Comparisons for Coping with Regrets Across Adulthood," *Personality and Social Psychology Bulletin* 37, no. 2 (2011): 215–28, https://pubmed.ncbi.nlm.nih.gov/21239595/.

3. Giorgio Coricelli et al., "Regret and Its Avoidance: A Neuroimaging Study of Choice Behavior," *Nature Neuroscience* 8 (2005): 1255–62, https://doi.org/10.1038/nn1514.

4. Roderick M. Chisholm, "The Contrary-to-Fact Conditional," *Mind* 55, no. 220 (1946): 289–307, https://www.jstor.org/stable/2250757.

5. Kai Epstude and Neal J. Roese, "The Functional Theory of Counterfactual Thinking," *Personal and Social Psychology Review* 12, no. 2 (2008): 168–92, https://psycnet.apa.org/record/2008-05743-004.

6. Parikh, de Brigard, and LaBar, "The Efficacy of Downward Counterfactual Thinking."

7. Parikh, de Brigard, and LaBar, "The Efficacy of Downward Counterfactual Thinking"; Epstude and Roese, "The Functional Theory of Counterfactual Thinking"; Daniel Kahneman and Dale T. Miller, "Norm Theory: Comparing Reality to Its Alternatives," *Psychological Review* 93, no. 2 (1986): 136–53, https://psycnet.apa.org/record/1986-21899-001.

8. Neal J. Roese and Amy Summerville, "What We Regret Most . . . and Why," *Personality and Social Psychology Review* 10, no. 3 (2006): 210–24, https://www.ncbi.nlm.nih.gov/pmc/articles/PMC2394712/.

9. Clemson University, "Practical Use for Regret, Hindsight," Science Daily, July 25, 2019, https://www.sciencedaily.com/releases/2019/07/190725162314.htm.

10. Susan Krauss Whitbourne, "Building Your Life Story: One Memory at a Time," *Psychology Today*, April 26, 2024, https://www.psychologytoday.com/us/blog/fulfillment-at-any-age/202404/building-your-life-story-one-memory-at-a-time.

11. Edward de Bono, *Six Thinking Hats*, rev. and updated ed. (Back Bay Books, 1999).

Chapter 12 Help, I Don't Know What the Heck Is Happening!

1. As quoted in "Quote: Paulos on Uncertainty," CAUSE, accessed January 15, 2025, https://www.causeweb.org/cause/resources/library/r2028.

2. Caroline Leaf, "Research," Dr. Leaf, accessed September 18, 2024, https://drleaf.com/pages/research-history.

Chapter 13 Help, My Past Is Haunting Me!

1. Centers for Disease Control and Prevention, "About Child Abuse and Neglect," CDC: Child Abuse and Neglect Prevention, accessed September 18, 2024, https://www.cdc.gov/child-abuse-neglect/about/index.html.

2. Idaho Youth Ranch, "Symptoms of Toxic Stress & Childhood PTSD," Idaho Youth Ranch, accessed December 9, 2024, https://www.youthranch.org/blog/childhood-ptsd-symptoms-of-toxic-stress.

3. Andy Turner, "Good Intentions but the Right Approach? The Case of ACEs," *Public Healthy* (blog), January 29, 2019, https://publichealthy.co.uk/good-intentions-but-the-right-approach-the-case-of-aces/.

4. Idaho Youth Ranch, "Childhood Trauma & Adverse Childhood Experiences," Idaho Youth Ranch, accessed December 9, 2024, https://www.youthranch.org/overview-childhood-trauma.

5. HOPE, "Positive Childhood Experiences and Adult Mental Health," HOPE—Healthy Outcomes from Positive Experiences, accessed December 9, 2024, https://positiveexperience.org/wp-content/uploads/2020/03/BRFShandout2-18.pdf.

6. Richard Sears, "Japanese Study Strengthens Link Between Childhood Adversity and Later Psychological Distress," Mad in America, June 6, 2024, https://www.madinamerica.com/2024/06/japanese-study-strengthens-link-between-childhood-adversity-and-later-psychological-distress/; Natsu Sasaki et al., "Effects of Expanded Adverse Childhood Experiences Including School Bullying, Childhood Poverty, and Natural Disasters on Mental Health in Adulthood," *Scientific Reports* 14, no. 1 (2024): 12015, https://doi.org/10.1038/s41598-024-62634-7.

7. Annie Wright, "Embracing Complexity: Was My Childhood Really That Bad?" *Psychology Today*, May 22, 2024, https://www.psychologytoday.com/us/blog/making-the-whole-beautiful/202405/embracing-complexity-was-my-childhood-really-that-bad.

8. Vanessa Villafuerte, "Study Reveals Types of Positive Childhood Experiences (PCEs) Linked to Improved Mental and Physical Health Outcomes in Adulthood," UCLA Health, December 8, 2023, https://www.uclahealth.org/news/release/study-reveals-types-positive-childhood-experiences-pces.

9. Villafuerte, "Study Reveals Types"; HOPE, "Positive Childhood Experiences."

10. HOPE, "Positive Childhood Experiences."

11. Vincent J. Felitti et al., "Relationship of Childhood Abuse and Household Dysfunction to Many of the Leading Causes of Death in Adults: The Adverse Childhood Experiences (ACE) Study," *American Journal of Preventive Medicine* 14, no. 4 (1998): 245–58, https://pubmed.ncbi.nlm.nih.gov/9635069/.

12. Gary Walsh, "The ACEs Campaign: Cause for Worry or Celebration?" *TES Magazine*, November 11, 2018, https://www.tes.com

/magazine/archive/aces-campaign-cause-worry-or-celebration. See also Turner, "Good Intentions but the Right Approach?"

13. Wright, "Embracing Complexity"; Turner, "Good Intentions but the Right Approach?"

14. Barbara Fredrickson, *Positivity: Top-Notch Research Reveals the 3-to-1 Ratio That Will Change Your Life* (Harmony, 2009); Michael A. Cohn et al., "Happiness Unpacked: Positive Emotions Increase Life Satisfaction by Building Resilience," *Emotion* 9, no. 3 (2009): 361–68, https://pmc.ncbi.nlm.nih.gov/articles/PMC3126102/; Barbara Fredrickson et al., "Open Hearts Build Lives: Positive Emotions, Induced Through Loving-Kindness Meditation, Build Consequential Personal Resources," *Journal of Personality and Social Psychology* 95, no. 5 (2008): 1045–62, https://pmc.ncbi.nlm.nih.gov/articles/PMC3156028/.

15. Caroline Leaf et al., "Psycho-Neuro-Biological Correlates of Beta Activity," *NeuroRegulation* 10, no. 1 (2023): 11–20, https://www.neuroregulation.org/article/view/23374/14748.

Chapter 14 Help, I'm a People Pleaser!

1. Fay Lane (@faera_lane), "Recovering people pleasers will be like 'I am in my . . .'" X post, June 17, 2022, https://x.com/faera_lane/status/1539085376320684032; Valentina Mejia, "I'm in My Villain Era. Here Are 5 Ways I Achieve the Look & Lifestyle," Refinery29, October 28, 2022, https://www.refinery29.com/en-us/2022/10/11167660/villain-era-tiktok-aesthetic-lifestyle.

Chapter 15 Help, My Inner Critic Won't Let Up!

1. David Muehsam et al., "The Embodied Mind: A Review on Functional Genomic and Neurological Correlates of Mind-Body Therapies," *Neuroscience and Behavioral Reviews* 73 (2017): 161–81, https://pubmed.ncbi.nlm.nih.gov/28017838/; Joao Freitas, "Teacher Shows Students How Negative Words Can Make Rice Moldy," Good News Network, June 11, 2017, https://www.goodnewsnetwork.org/teacher-shows-students-how-negative-words-makes-rice-moldy/.

Chapter 16 Help, I'm Self-Diagnosing Again!

1. Ellen McVay, "Social Media and Self-Diagnosis," Johns Hopkins All Children's Hospital, August 31, 2023, https://www.hopkinsmedicine.org/news/articles/2023/08/social-media-and-self-diagnosis.

2. Afton M. Koball et al., "Distress Tolerance and Psychological Comorbidity in Patients Seeking Bariatric Surgery," *Obesity Surgery* 26, no. 7 (2016): 1559–64, https://pubmed.ncbi.nlm.nih.gov/26464243/.

3. Lucy Foulkes and Jack L. Andrews, "Are Mental Health Awareness Efforts Contributing to the Rise in Reported Mental Health Problems? A Call to Test the Prevalence Inflation Hypothesis," *New Ideas in Psychology* 69 (2023): 101010, https://www.sciencedirect.com/science/article/pii/S0732118X2300003X.

4. ScienceDirect, "Mental Health," ScienceDirect Topics, accessed September 18, 2024, https://www.sciencedirect.com/topics/psychology/mental-health.

5. Ellen Barry, "Are We Talking Too Much About Mental Health?," *New York Times*, May 6, 2024, https://www.nytimes.com/2024/05/06/health/mental-health-schools.html.

6. Zoe Cunniffe, "The TikTokification of Mental Health on Campus," Mad in America, June 22, 2024, https://www.madinamerica.com/2024/06/the-tiktokification-of-mental-health-on-campus/.

7. "Best Mentalhealthawareness TikTok Hashtags," TikTok Hashtags, accessed September 18, 2024, https://tiktokhashtags.com/hashtag/mentalhealthawareness/; Sultana Ismet Jerin, Nicole O'Donnell, and Di Mu, "Mental Health Messages on TikTok: Analysing the Use of Emotional Appeals in Health-Related #EduTok Videos," *Health Education Journal* 83 no. 4 (2024): 395–408, https://doi.org/10.1177/00178969241235528.

8. Cunniffe, "The TikTokification of Mental Health on Campus."

9. Howard N. Garb, "Race Bias and Gender Bias in the Diagnosis of Psychological Disorders," *Clinical Psychology Review* 90 (2021): 102087, https://www.sciencedirect.com/science/article/abs/pii/S0272735821001306.

10. Margarita Panayiotou et al., "Time Spent on Social Media Among the Least Influential Factors in Adolescent Mental Health: Preliminary Results from a Panel Network Analysis," *Nature Mental Health* 1 (2023): 316–26, https://doi.org/10.1038/s44220-023-00063-7.

11. Brian TaeHyuk Keum et al., "Benefits and Harms of Social Media Use: A Latent Profile Analysis of Emerging Adults," *Current Psychology* 42, no. 9 (2022): 1–13, https://www.ncbi.nlm.nih.gov/pmc/articles/PMC9302950/.

12. Liz Do, "Is Social Media Fueling the Youth Mental Health Crisis?" UCI School of Social Ecology, August 25, 2023, https://socialecology.uci.edu/news/social-media-fueling-youth-mental-health-crisis; Candice L. Odgers, "The Panic Over Smartphones Doesn't Help Teens," *Atlantic*, May 21, 2024, https://www.theatlantic.com/technology/archive/2024/05/candice-odgers-teens-smartphones/678433/?utm_source=apple_news.

13. Candice L. Odgers and Michaeline Jensen, "Annual Research Review: Adolescent Mental Health in the Digital Age: Facts, Fears, and Future Directions," *Journal of the American Academy of Child & Adolescent Psychiatry* 61, no. 3 (2020): 336–48, https://pubmed.ncbi.nlm.nih.gov/31951670/.

14. Odgers, "The Panic Over Smartphones Doesn't Help Teens."

Chapter 17 Help, Technology Is Everywhere!

1. Serena Baudacco et al., "A Bidirectional Model of Sleep and Technology Use: A Theoretical Review of How Much, for Whom, and Which Mechanisms," *Sleep Medicine Reviews* 76 (2024): 101933, https://www.sciencedirect.com/science/article/pii/S1087079224000376?mod=ANLink.

2. Baudacco et al., "Bidirectional Model"; Melinda Beck, "Open the Book, Put Down the Tablet at Bedtime," *Wall Street Journal*, December 22, 2014, https://www.wsj.com/articles/open-the-book-close-the-e-reader-at-bedtime-1419272534?mod=ANLink.

3. Xanne Janssen et al., "Associations of Screen Time, Sedentary Time and Physical Activity with Sleep in Under 5s: A Systematic Review and Meta-Analysis," *Sleep Medicine Reviews* 49 (2020): 101226, https://www.sciencedirect.com/science/article/pii/S1087079219301947; Lisbeth Lund et al., "Electronic Media Use and Sleep in Children and Adolescents in Western Countries: A Systematic Review," *BMC Public Health* 21 (2021): 1598, https://doi.org/10.1186/s12889-021-11640-9.

4. Alex Janin, "Screen Time Before Bed Might Not Be That Bad After All," *Wall Street Journal*, May 29, 2024, https://www.wsj.com/health/wellness/sleep-blue-light-screens-dbb796e7.

5. Janin, "Screen Time Before Bed."

6. Baudacco et al., "Bidirectional Model."

7. Brian Stelter, "8 Hours a Day Spent on Screens, Study Finds," *New York Times*, March 26, 2009, https://www.nytimes.com/2009/03/27/business/media/27adco.html.

Chapter 18 Help, Everything Is Going Wrong!

1. Morgan Harper Nichols, *Peace Is a Practice: An Invitation to Breathe Deep and Find a New Rhythm for Life*, Kindle ed. (Zondervan, 2022), 2.

2. Sophie Vandepitte et al., "The Role of 'Peace of Mind' and 'Meaningfulness' as Psychological Concepts in Explaining Subjective Well-Being," *Journal of Happiness Studies* 23 (2022): 3331–46, https://doi.org/10.1007/s10902-022-00544-z; Michele Vecchione et al., "The Associations Between Grandiose Narcissism and Perfectionism: New Insights Into an Old Debate," *Personality and Individual Differences* 215 (2023): 112395, https://doi.org/10.1016/j.paid.2023.112395; Leaf et al., "Habit Formation and Automaticity"; Leaf et al., "Psycho-Neuro-Biological Correlates of Beta Activity."

3. James A. Dungan, Michael Stepanovic, and Liane Young, "Theory of Mind for Processing Unexpected Events Across Contexts," *Social Cognitive and Affective Neuroscience* 11, no. 8 (2016): 1183–92, https://doi.org/10.1093/scan/nsw032.

4. Guy William Fincham et al., "Effect of Breathwork on Stress and Mental Health: A Meta-Analysis of Randomised-Controlled Trials," *Scientific Reports* 13 (2023): 432, https://doi.org/10.1038/s41598-022-27247-y.

5. Andrea Zaccaro et al., "How Breath-Control Can Change Your Life: A Systematic Review on Psycho-Physiological Correlates of Slow Breathing," *Frontiers in Human Neuroscience* 12 (2018): 353, https://doi.org/10.3389/fnhum.2018.00353.

6. Divya Budhraja Mathur, "My Favorite Team Building Activity: On Asking for Help," *Eat Teach Blog* (blog), April 25, 2018, https://eatteachblog.com/team-building-activity/.

7. Amy Morin, "7 Scientifically Proven Benefits of Gratitude," *Psychology Today*, April 3, 2015, https://www.psychologytoday.com/us/blog/what-mentally-strong-people-dont-do/201504/7-scientifically-proven-benefits-gratitude.

8. Morin, "7 Scientifically Proven Benefits."

9. *Oxford Reference*, "Maya Angelou 1928–2014," accessed September 24, 2024, https://www.oxfordreference.com/display/10.1093/acref/9780191866692.001.0001/q-oro-ed6-00000286.

Conclusion

1. "Sam Sundquist Quotes," Goodreads, accessed September 18, 2024, https://www.goodreads.com/quotes/579286-some-days-you-just-have-to-create-your-own-sunshine.

2. Courtney Sembler, "A Bad Day Not a Bad Life," Medium, April 16, 2019, https://medium.com/@CSembler/a-bad-day-not-a-bad-life-ea02fabd2faf.

3. "Slow Progress Is Better Than No Progress," Pinterest pin, posted by Look Up Quotes, accessed September 18, 2024, https://ie.pinterest.com/pin/slow-progress-is-better-than-no-progress--556687203949408126/.

4. "Oh Yes, the Past Can Hurt," Pinterest pin, posted by Reyton Santos, accessed September 18, 2024, https://br.pinterest.com/pin/194499277644042847/.

5. "Brendon Burchard Quotes," BrainyQuote, accessed September 18, 2024, https://www.brainyquote.com/quotes/brendon_burchard_864738.

6. "Bernie S. Siegel Quotes," Goodreads, accessed September 18, 2024, https://www.goodreads.com/author/quotes/683.Bernie_S_Siegel.

7. "Gregory S. Williams Quotes," Goodreads, accessed September 18, 2024, https://www.goodreads.com/author/quotes/6491152.Gregory_S_Williams.

8. Larry Lewis, "Turn Your Wounds into Wisdom," *Larry Lewis* (blog), accessed September 18, 2024, https://www.larry-lewis.com/5381/turn-your-wounds-into-wisdom.

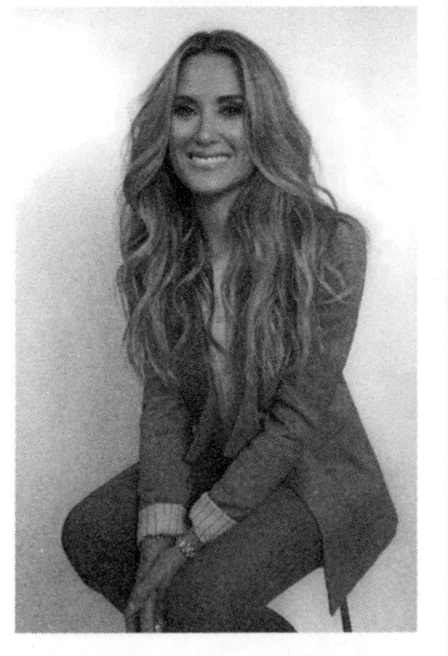

DR. CAROLINE LEAF

is a communication pathologist and clinical neuroscientist specializing in psychoneurobiology. Her passion is to help people see the power of the mind to change the brain, control chaotic thinking, and find mental peace. She is the author of several bestselling books, including *Cleaning Up Your Mental Mess*, *Switch On Your Brain*, *How to Help Your Child Clean Up Their Mental Mess*, *Think and Eat Yourself Smart*, *The Perfect You*, and *Think, Learn, Succeed*. She is also host of the top-rated podcast *Cleaning Up the Mental Mess*, which has over forty million downloads. She currently does extensive research and teaches at various academic, medical, corporate, and neuroscience conferences, as well as in religious and spiritual institutions around the world. Dr. Leaf and her husband, Mac, have four adult children and live in Cleveland, Ohio.

Connect with Caroline:

DrLeaf.com

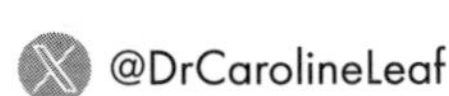

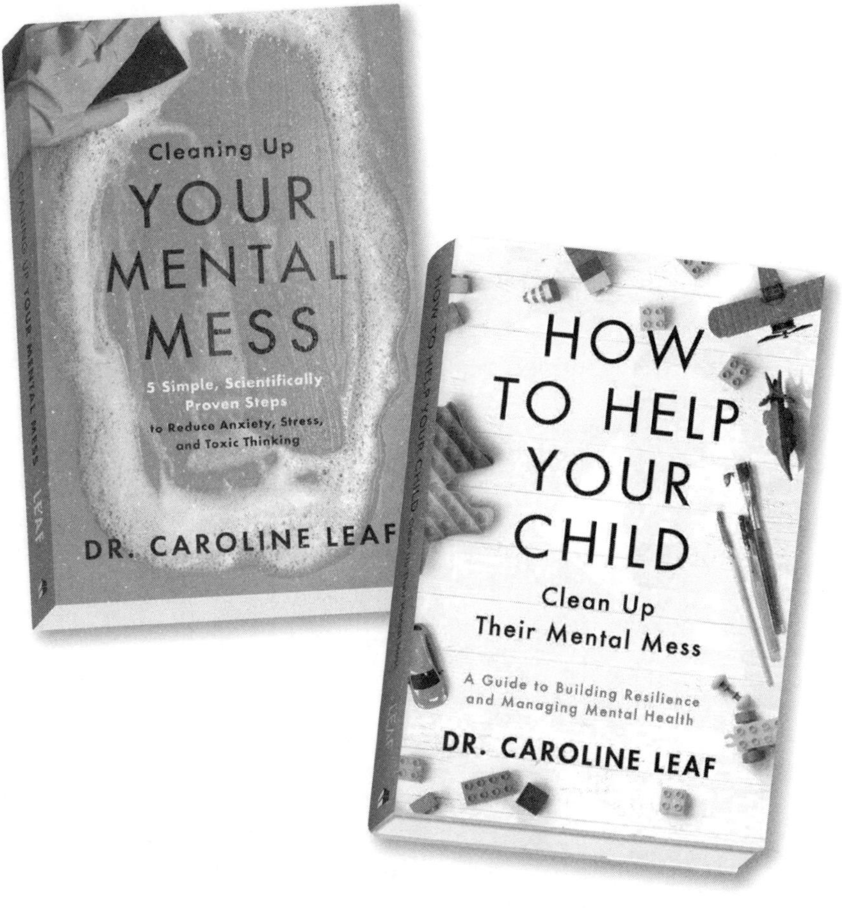

Connect with
CAROLINE

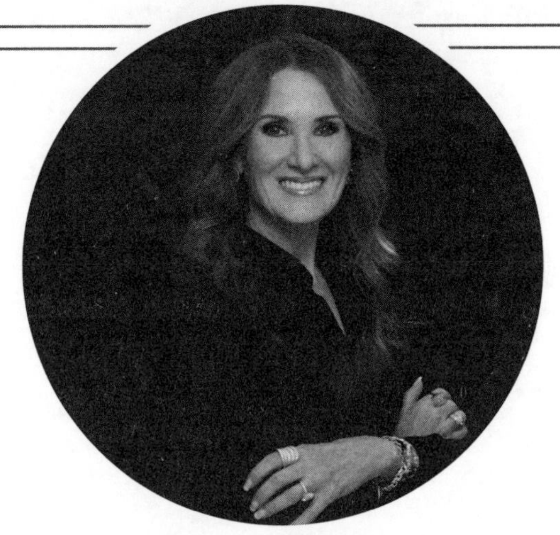

VISIT

DrLeaf.com

to learn more about Dr. Leaf and her research, read her blog, listen to her podcast, and follow her speaking schedule!

Also follow her on social media.

drleaf

DrCarolineLeaf

drcarolineleaf

Dr. Caroline Leaf

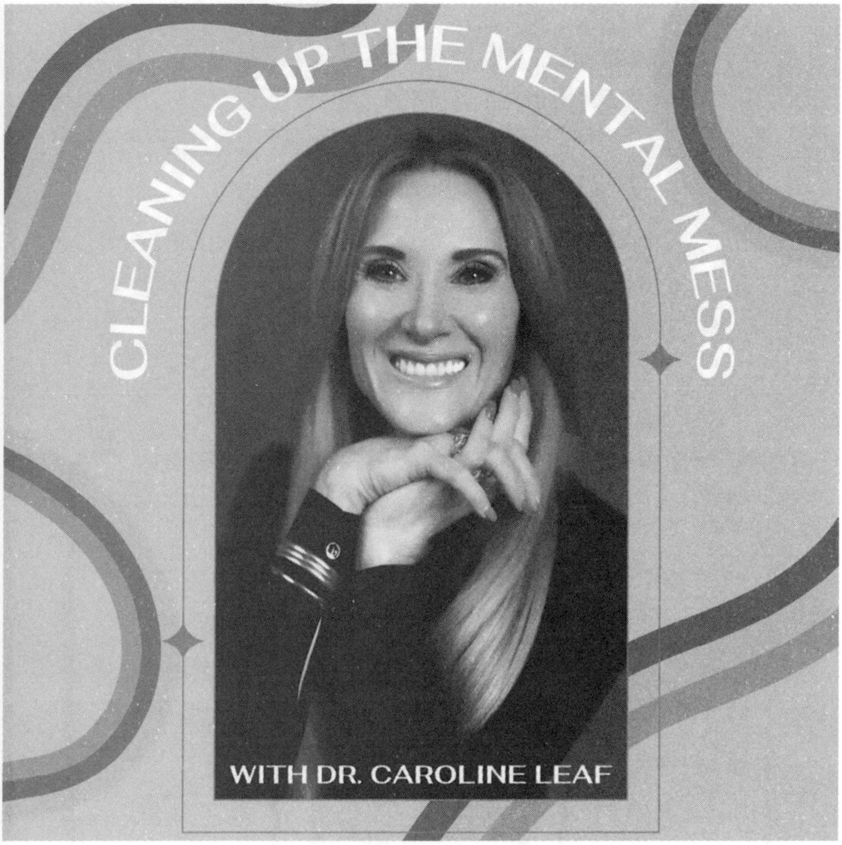